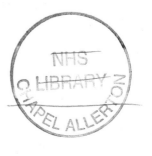

An Atlas of
SCHIZOPHRENIA

The presentation of this copy has
been made possible by an
unrestricted educational grant from

 Bristol-Myers Squibb

and

 Otsuka Pharmaceuticals

Advancing Science in Psychiatry

THE ENCYCLOPEDIA OF VISUAL MEDICINE SERIES

An Atlas of
SCHIZOPHRENIA

Martin Stefan
Fulbourn Hospital, Cambridge, UK

Mike Travis
Institute of Psychiatry, De Crespigny Park, London, UK

and

Robin M. Murray
Institute of Psychiatry, De Crespigny Park, London, UK

The Parthenon Publishing Group
International Publishers in Medicine, Science & Technology

A CRC PRESS COMPANY
BOCA RATON   LONDON   NEW YORK   WASHINGTON, D.C.

Published in the UK and Europe by
The Parthenon Publishing Group
23–25 Blades Court
Deodar Road
London, SW15 2NU, UK

Published in the USA by
The Parthenon Publishing Group
345 Park Avenue South, 10th Floor
New York 10010, USA

Library of Congress Cataloging-in-Publication Data
An atlas of schizophrenia / [edited by] Martin Stefan, Mike Travis and Robin M. Murray.
       p. ; cm. -- (Encyclopedia of visual medicine series)
   Includes bibliographical references and index.
   ISBN 1-85070-074-5 (alk. paper)
     1. Schizophrenia -- Atlases. I. Stefan, Martin. II. Travis, Mike. III. Murray, Robin MD,
MPhil, MRCP, MRCPsych. IV. Series.
       [DNLM: 1. Schizophrenia--Atlases. WM 17 A8813 2001]
   RC514 A86 2001
   616.89'82--dc21
                                                                                         2001052033

British Library Cataloguing in Publication Data
An atlas of schizophrenia. - (The encyclopedia of visual medicine series)
   1. Schizophrenia
   I. Stefan, Martin II. Travis, Mike III. Murray, Robin, 1944-
   616.8'982
   ISBN 1850700745

Composition by The Parthenon Publishing Group, London, UK
Color reproduction by Graphic Reproductions, Morecambe, UK
Printed and bound by T. G. Hostench S. A., Spain

Contents

Other atlases in this series include:

Epilepsy
Parkinson's Disease
Multiple Sclerosis
Headache
Stroke
Depression
Pain
Prostatic Diseases
Erectile Dysfunction
Hair and Scalp Disorders
Gastroenterology
Sigmoidoscopy and Cytoscopy
Diabetes
Uro-oncology

Preface

There have been major changes in attitudes towards schizophrenia in recent years. In clinical practice, more effective pharmacological and psychological treatments for schizophrenia have helped regenerate a sense of therapeutic optimism. In research, progress in a range of basic disciplines has opened up new avenues which promise to help unravel the abnormalities of brain development, structure and function which are at the core of the disorder. These have been complimented by advances from epidemiology which remind us that schizophrenia is not just a brain disorder, and that social and psychological factors can have a profound impact on its onset and outcome. Research in schizophrenia has never been more exciting. This Atlas is our attempt to put together a visual overview of this fascinating and challenging territory.

We have included many of the more familiar landmarks and monuments, but also some informative images of the most interesting new developments. Inevitably, because of the vast volume of new developments, our compilation has been somewhat selective. However, we hope this Atlas reflects our sense that a cohesive clinical and theoretical understanding of this complex disorder is now within reach, and that we can now bring hope and better care to sufferers.

Martin Stefan, Mike Travis
and Robin M. Murray
November 2001

Foreword

Schizophrenia is a puzzle. Emil Kraepelin considered that his life's work had resulted merely in progress in understanding the psychoses, not a solution. Gottesman and Shields regarded the causes of schizophrenia as being an epigenetic puzzle, an analogy that continues to serve us well. Research in this area seems to produce ever more pieces, rather than fitting them together.

More importantly, schizophrenia puzzles patients who have the syndrome, their families and, as often as not, the clinicians who try to help them. Martin Stefan, Mike Travis and Robin Murray are experts in this field, and have produced an excellent and highly readable overview of the clinical features of the disorder, the epidemiological context, possible causes, and the current status of drug treatment. Clinicians working in all aspects of services for people with schizophrenia will find this an accessible and clear reference. Many may consider recommending the book to some patients and carers who want

rather more information than is contained in standard educational materials.

An atlas is probably not the most obvious format for a book on schizophrenia but the authors have succeeded in producing a useful and interesting one. Diagrams, tables and figures give contemporary views an immediate impact, with modern techniques of investigation, such as neuroimaging, being particularly well suited to this format. These are balanced by the paintings from the Bethlem Royal Hospital Archives and Museum that entertain and fascinate alongside the factual information: they give an impression of the human as well as scientific and psychiatric aspects of schizophrenia. Thus, the book provides a useful map for all.

Peter Jones
Professor of Psychiatry
University of Cambridge

CHAPTER 1

Clinical features

HISTORY AND CLASSIFICATION

Schizophrenia is arguably the most severe of the psychiatric disorders. It carries a lifetime risk of around 0.5–1%, and its early onset and tendency to chronicity mean that its prevalence is relatively high. Disability results particularly from negative symptoms and cognitive deficits, features that can have a greater impact on long-term functioning than the more dramatic delusions and hallucinations which often characterize relapses. The social and economic impact of the illness is enormous, and its impact on sufferers and their families can be devastating.

Although descriptions of people who may have had schizophrenia-like illnesses can be found throughout history (Figure 1.1) the first comprehensive descriptions date from the beginning of the 18th century (Figures 1.2 and 1.3)[1]. The modern concept of schizophrenia was first formalized by the German psychiatrist Emil Kraepelin (Figure 1.4)[2,3] at the turn of the 20th century. Kraepelin, who drew on contemporary accounts of syndromes such as catatonia and hebephrenia, was the first to distinguish between

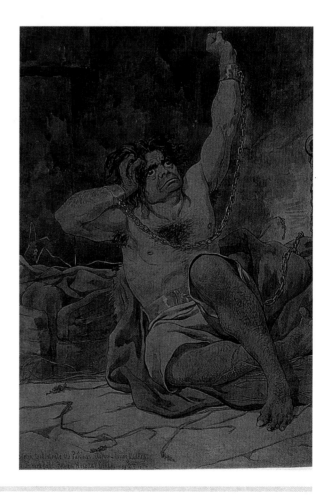

Figure 1.1 Sketch to Illustrate the Passions: Agony – Raving Madness, by Richard Dadd (1854). In this painting, Richard Dadd (1817–1886) alludes to a pre-Kraeplinian distinction between 'raving madness' and 'melancholic madness'. Dadd himself was a patient at the Bethlem (Bedlam) Hospital, England's oldest mental hospital, and at Broadmoor, the hospital for the criminally insane. A Victorian painter best known for his fairy paintings, Dadd developed his illness at around the age of 25, when he become suspicious and preoccupied with religion, and developed delusions relating to the Egyptian god Assyris, beliefs that thoughts and commands which he had to obey were put into his head, and delusions that he was persecuted by the devil. At the age of 27, in response to these beliefs, he attacked and killed his father. He spent the rest of his life in institutional psychiatric care. Figure reproduced with kind permission of the Bethlem Royal Hospital Archives and Museum, Beckenham, Kent, UK

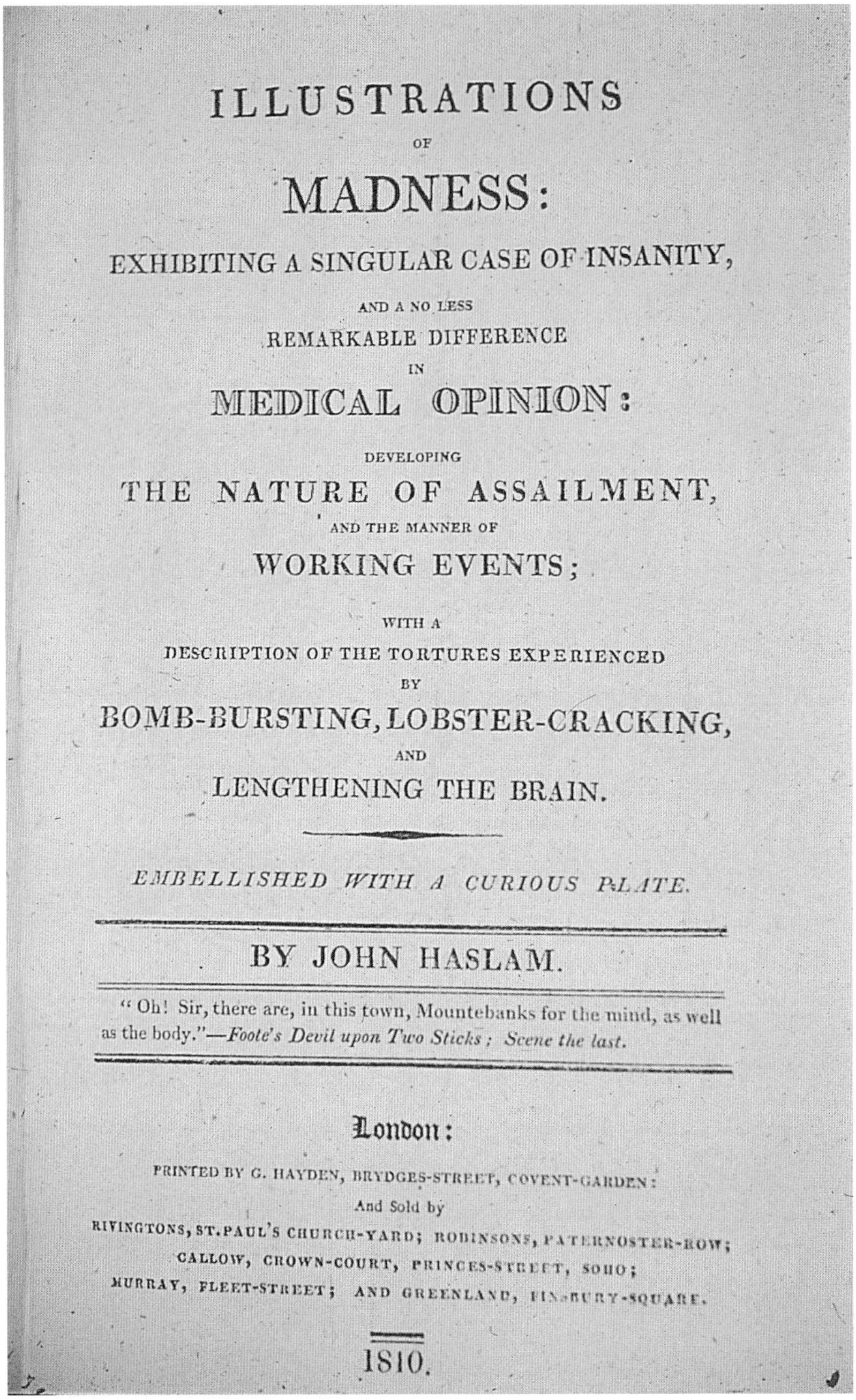

ILLUSTRATIONS

OF

MADNESS:

EXHIBITING A SINGULAR CASE OF INSANITY,

AND A NO LESS

REMARKABLE DIFFERENCE

IN

MEDICAL OPINION:

DEVELOPING

THE NATURE OF ASSAILMENT,

AND THE MANNER OF

WORKING EVENTS;

WITH A

DESCRIPTION OF THE TORTURES EXPERIENCED

BY

BOMB-BURSTING, LOBSTER-CRACKING,

AND

LENGTHENING THE BRAIN.

EMBELLISHED WITH A CURIOUS PLATE.

BY JOHN HASLAM.

" Oh! Sir, there are, in this town, Mountebanks for the mind, as well as the body."—*Foote's Devil upon Two Sticks; Scene the last.*

London:

PRINTED BY G. HAYDEN, BRYDGES-STREET, COVENT-GARDEN:

And Sold by

RIVINGTONS, ST. PAUL'S CHURCH-YARD; ROBINSONS, PATERNOSTER-ROW;

CALLOW, CROWN-COURT, PRINCES-STREET, SOHO;

MURRAY, FLEET-STREET; AND GREENLAND, FINSBURY-SQUARE.

1810.

Figure 1.2 Frontispiece from Illustrations of Madness (1810), by John Haslam[1], which provides a vivid description of psychosis in an individual patient early in the industrial revolution. James Tilley Matthews was admitted to the Bethlem Hospital in 1797, after writing a threatening letter to a senior official in the British Admiralty. Haslam, who was Matthews' doctor at the Bethlem, wrote his book as a rebuttal of claims made in court that Matthews was not insane. Matthews believed that a 'gang of villains, profoundly skilled in pneumatic chemistry' were assailing him: 'while one of these villains is sucking out the brain of the person assailed, to extract his existing sentiments, another of the gang will force into his mind a train of ideas very different from the real subject of his thoughts'. He experienced many other unpleasant experiences, including 'sudden death squeezing, stomach skinning, apoplexy making with the nutmeg grater, lengthening of the brain, thought making and laugh making'. Figure reproduced with kind permission of the Bethlem Royal Hospital Archives and Museum, Beckenham, Kent, UK

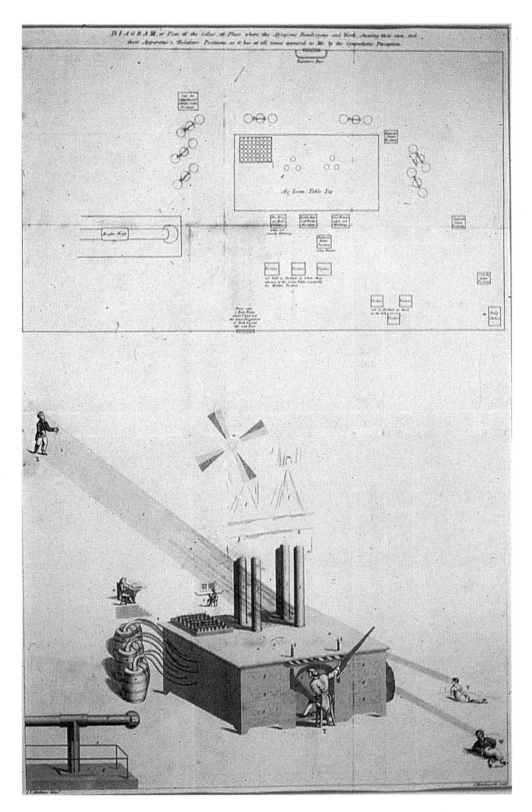

Figure 1.3 Air-loom, by James Tilley Matthews, circa 1810. This plate is included in Haslam's book[1]. It is Matthews' own 'diagram or plan of the cellar or place where the assassins rendezvous and work, showing their own and their apparatuses' relative positions, as it has at all times appeared to me by the sympathetic perception'. As well as the 'air-loom', Matthews indicates the sources of various abnormal experiences: the voices of the King, Bill, the Middle Man, the Glove Woman, Augusta, Charlotte, St Archy, and assorted visitors, who are 'not half so distinct as when they advance to the Loom Table, especially the Middle Position', together with a 'door into a back room where I have not the least perception of them beyond the said door'. Figure reproduced with kind permission of the Bethlem Royal Hospital Archives and Museum, Beckenham, Kent, UK

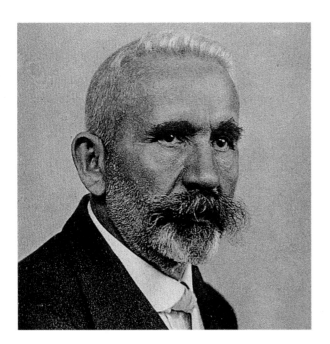

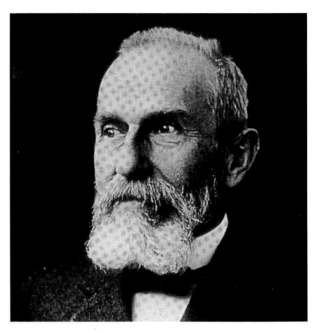

Figure 1.4 Emil Kraepelin (1856–1926). The fifth edition of Kraepelin's *Textbook of Psychiatry*[2], published in 1896, articulated a distinction between acquired and constitutional pathology in mental illness. The sixth edition, published in 1899, distinguished between dementia praecox and manic depressive insanity

Figure 1.5 Eugen Bleuler (1857–1939). In 1911, Eugen Bleuler published his monograph entitled *Dementia Praecox, or the Group of Schizophrenias*, and argued that dementia praecox was not a single disease, was not inevitably associated with intellectual decline, and had as its fundamental basis disorders of affectivity, ambivalence, autism, attention and will. Other symptoms such as delusions, hallucinations, abnormal behavior and catatonia were conceptualized as secondary 'accessory symptoms'

the two major poles of severe mental illness. He described one group of patients in whom the clinical picture was dominated by disordered mood and who followed a cyclical pattern of relapse and relative remission; he termed this 'manic depressive insanity'. Others had a deteriorating illness characterized by florid onset, often in adolescence, with a prolonged course marked by profound social and functional disability. He called the latter 'dementia praecox', and saw it as 'a single morbid process', endogenous rather than acquired, starting in youth and with dementia as a common outcome. This concept has since been enormously influential in guiding our perception of the disorder, even though Kraepelin himself came to recognize many of its limitations: for example, the disease was not always confined to younger people, the progression to dementia was not inevitable and in some individuals a recovery would be seen[4].

The Swiss psychiatrist Eugen Bleuler (Figure 1.5) coined the term 'schizophrenia' in 1911 and this rapidly displaced dementia praecox[5]. Unlike Kraepelin, who was strongly influenced by the successes of clinical pathology in the search for causative agents in diseases such as syphilis and tuberculosis, Bleuler thought of schizophrenia in psychological rather than neuropathological terms. For Bleuler, the florid but highly variable symptoms of psychosis, such as delusions and hallucinations, were secondary, 'accessory' phenomena. At the core of the illness, he believed, was a more generalized psychological deficit, characterised by a 'loosening of associations' in the form of language, by deficits in volition and attention, and by incongruity of affect, ambivalence and autism.

Although intellectually compelling as a model of schizophrenia, Bleuler's core symptoms were difficult to define reliably. In particular, the limits

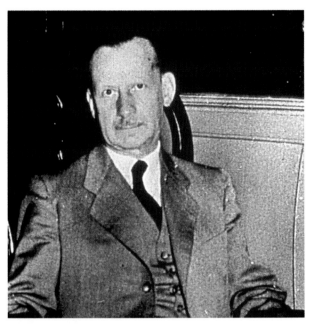

SCHNEIDER'S SYMPTOMS OF THE FIRST RANK

- Audible thoughts
- Voices heard arguing
- Voices heard commenting on one's actions
- The experience of influences playing on the body
- Thought withdrawal and other interferences with thought
- Diffusion of thought
- Delusional perception
- Feelings, impulses and volitional acts experienced as the work or influence of others

Figure 1.6 Kurt Schneider. In 1959 he listed the 'first rank features' of schizophrenia. One of these symptoms, in the absence of organic disease, persistent affective disorder, or drug intoxication, was sufficient for a diagnosis of schizophrenia

of 'simple schizophrenia' (schizophrenia uncomplicated by 'accessory' symptoms) and 'latent schizophrenia' (people with odd personalities said to share some of the characteristics of the full-blown disorder) were difficult to define. This confusion was compounded by the clinical heterogeneity of schizophrenia, the lack of clear prognostic features and the failure to discover any definitive pathological abnormalities, and led to an expansion of the concept of schizophrenia to the extent that it became a vague synonym for severe mental illness with different meanings in different countries. This was especially the case in the USA, where Bleuler's concepts held great sway, and in the former Soviet Union, where different models (incorporating, for example, anorexia nervosa sufferers and political dissenters) had developed.

In Western Europe, where the Kraeplinian formulation remained dominant, diagnosis was more consistent, partly because the positive psychotic symptoms central to the Kraeplinian definition are more readily and reliably determined. In 1959[6], Kurt Schneider (Figure 1.6) set out a list of such symptoms, which would be most likely, in the absence of organic brain disease, to

lead to the diagnosis of schizophrenia. These 'symptoms of the first rank' were selected because they were relatively easily elicited and reliably identified, rather than because of any central theoretical importance; nevertheless, they were highly influential in determining diagnostic practice.

The International Pilot Study of Schizophrenia[7] (IPSS; Figure 1.7) which investigated the illness in several centers around the world, suggested a high degree of consistency in the clinical picture of schizophrenia when diagnosed using strict diagnostic rules. This appeared to hold true in rural and in urban areas, and both in Western European countries and in developing countries. The use of operationalized diagnostic rules in this, and in the earlier US/UK Diagnostic Project, greatly facilitated research into the epidemiology of the disorder. Since then, as a result of the development and use of operationalized definitions in the *Diagnostic and Statistical Manual*[8] *of Mental Disorders* (DSM–IV) in the USA, and the *International Classification of Diseases*[9] (ICD–10) worldwide, definitions of schizophrenia have been considerably narrowed.

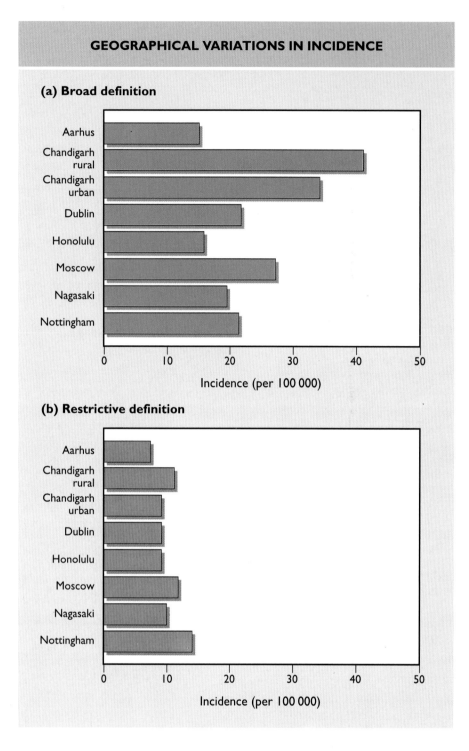

Figure 1.7 Geographical variations in the incidence of schizophrenia, (a) broadly defined and (b) narrowly defined. These data from the International Pilot Study of Schizophrenia[7] were taken as evidence that, particularly when narrow operational criteria are used, the incidence of schizophrenia is remarkably constant between countries. Although this was very influential when it was published, subsequent studies have demonstrated that the incidence does indeed vary, with higher rates found in those born or brought up in cities and in certain immigrant groups

Although diagnosis still depends on the presence of combinations of symptoms and the course of illness, and diagnostic practice may vary to some extent from country to country, there is a core group of patients who fulfill all definitions and would be diagnosed as suffering from schizophrenia anywhere in the world (Figure 1.8).

Both ICD–10 and DSM–IV identify a number of subtypes of schizophrenia. In clinical practice, a distinction is also often made between acute and chronic schizophrenia. A third way of thinking about the varied clinical picture seen in schizophrenia is in terms of syndromes (Figure 1.9). Unlike subtypes, syndromes do not

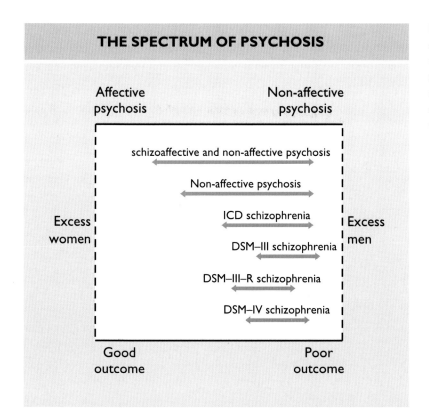

THE SPECTRUM OF PSYCHOSIS

Affective psychosis   Non-affective psychosis

schizoaffective and non-affective psychosis

Non-affective psychosis

ICD schizophrenia

DSM–III schizophrenia

DSM–III–R schizophrenia

DSM–IV schizophrenia

Excess women   Excess men

Good outcome   Poor outcome

Figure 1.8 Despite the advent of a variety of operational definitions, categorical definitions of schizophrenia vary in their cut-off points on a theoretical continuum. However, there is substantial overlap between diagnostic systems and a significant proportion of patients fulfil criteria in all systems

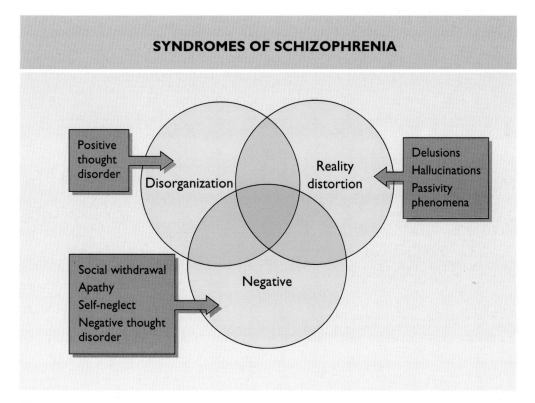

SYNDROMES OF SCHIZOPHRENIA

Positive thought disorder

Disorganization

Reality distortion

Delusions
Hallucinations
Passivity phenomena

Social withdrawal
Apathy
Self-neglect
Negative thought disorder

Negative

Figure 1.9 Symptoms of schizophrenia appear to cluster into three syndromes: 'positive', or reality distortion, characterized by delusions and hallucinations; 'negative', consisting of the 'deficit' symptoms including 'negative thought disorder', such as poverty of speech and poverty of content of speech; and 'disorganization', in which 'positive' formal thought disorder, for example knight's move thinking or loosening of associations are seen

represent exclusive domains; any individual patient may have features of more than one syndrome. Initial syndromal studies distinguished between positive and negative symptoms, but more recent work using factor-analytic studies of associations between symptoms supports the existence of a third syndrome, characterized by positive thought disorder or 'disorganization'. Thus, most clinicians would recognize the existence of psychotic symptom clusters in the following three domains:

1. Delusions and hallucinations, the so-called 'positive' symptoms.

2. Positive thought disorder or 'disorganization'.

3. Social withdrawal, apathy, self-neglect, poverty of speech and of content of speech, and other broadly 'negative' symptoms.

CLINICAL PRESENTATION AND SYMPTOMATOLOGY

As in the rest of medicine, reliable diagnosis depends on accurate history taking and clinical examination. The family and personal history may offer important etiological clues. There may be a family history of schizophrenia, complications in pregnancy or birth, or a personal history of childhood problems. Recent studies, including the follow-up of the British 1946 birth cohort[10], have suggested that children who later develop schizophrenia are more likely to have a history of developmental delay, as well as slightly lower IQ and educational achievements than other children (Figure 1.10). They are also more likely to have interpersonal and behavioral difficulties. Mothers may describe their pre-morbid personality as having shown emotional detachment; 'preschizophrenic' children may appear cold and aloof, avoiding play and engaging in solitary occupations. Some may be prone to temper tantrums, tend to avoid competition, have odd ideas and seek refuge in fantasy. These characteristics are also over-represented in the families of schizophrenics, although they do not reliably predict the development of schizophrenia.

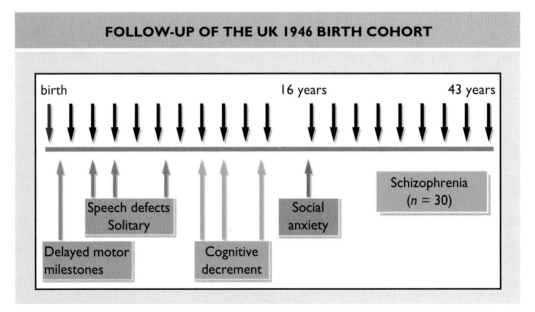

Figure 1.10 Differences between children destined to develop schizophrenia as adults and the general population were found across a range of developmental domains. As with some other adult illnesses, the origins of schizophrenia may be found in early life. This figure illustrates the associations between adult-onset schizophrenia and childhood sociodemographic, neurodevelopmental, cognitive, and behavioral factors in a cohort of 5362 people born in one week in 1946. Thirty cases of schizophrenia arose between ages 16 and 43 years. Data with permission from Jones P, Rodgers B, Murray R, et al. Child development risk factors for adult schizophrenia in the British 1946 birth cohort. Lancet 1994;344:1398–1402

DIFFERENTIAL DIAGNOSIS OF SCHIZOPHRENIA

'Functional'

Schizotypal disorder

Persistent delusional disorders

Acute and transient psychotic disorders

Schizoaffective disorders

Induced delusional disorder

Mania

Other nonorganic psychotic disorders

'Organic'

Drug/substance-induced psychosis (e.g. alcohol withdrawal, amphetamines, crack cocaine, LSD, cannabis, PCP, and also steroids, dopamine agonists and some heavy metals)

Epilepsy – in particular, the fits of temporal lobe epilepsy may resemble an acute psychotic episode

Tumors, either primary or secondary

Stroke

Early dementia

Long-term sequelae of head injury

Endocrine causes (e.g. Cushing's disease; rarely hyper- and hypothyroidism)

Infections (e.g. encephalitis, meningitis, neurosyphilis)

Multiple sclerosis

Autoimmune disorders such as systemic lupus erythematosus (SLE)

Metabolic disorders (e.g. hepatic failure, uremia, hypercalcemia, acute intermittent porphyria)

HALLUCINATIONS

Hallucinations are defined as false perceptions in the absence of a real external stimulus. They are perceived as having the same quality as real perceptions and are not usually subject to conscious manipulation.

Hallucinations in schizophrenia may involve any of the sensory modalities. The most common are auditory hallucinations in the form of voices, which occur in 60–70% of patients diagnosed with schizophrenia. Although voices in the second person are most common, the characteristic 'Schneiderian' voices are in the third person and provide a running commentary on the patient's actions, arguing about the patient or repeating the patient's thoughts. Voices may be imperative, ordering the patient to harm himself or others. Visual hallucinations occur in about 10% of patients, but should make one suspicious of an organic disorder. Olfactory hallucinations are more common in temporal lobe epilepsy than schizophrenia, and tactile hallucinations are probably experienced more frequently than is reported by patients.

No single type of hallucination is specific to schizophrenia, and the duration and intensity are probably most important diagnostically.

CATATONIC SYMPTOMS

These mainly motor symptoms may occur in any form of schizophrenia but are particularly associated with the catatonic subtype

Ambitendence Alternation between opposite movements.

Echopraxia Automatic imitation of another person's movements even when asked not to.

Stereotypies Repeated regular fixed parts of movement (or speech) that are not goal directed, e.g. moving the arm backwards and outwards repeatedly while saying 'but not for me'.

Negativism Motiveless resistance to instructions and attempts to be moved, or doing the opposite of what is asked.

Posturing Adoption of inappropriate or bizarre bodily posture continuously for a substantial period of time.

Waxy flexibility The patient's limbs can be 'molded' into a position and remain fixed for long periods of time.

THOUGHT DISORDERS

Usually a disorder of the form of thought, such that the speech is difficult to follow or incoherent and follows no logical sequence.

Knight's move thinking (or derailment) occurs when the patient moves from one train of thought to another which has no apparent connection to the first – it takes its name from the chess piece that moves two steps forward and one to the side. A less severe form is called **loosening of associations** which merges into **tangential thinking** and **loss of goal**.

Some patients may invent **neologisms** (new words), exhibit **verbal stereotypy** (repetition of a single word or phrase out of context), or use **metonyms** (ordinary words given a special personal meaning).

Negative thought disorder includes **poverty of speech** (limited quantity of speech), and poverty of content of speech (limited meaning conveyed by speech).

DISORDERS OF THOUGHT POSSESSION

Disorders of thought possession in schizophrenia are sometimes called thought alienation. The patient has the experience that his thoughts are under the control of an outside agency or that others are participating in his thinking.

Thought insertion The patient believes that thoughts that are not his own are being put into his mind by an external agency.

Thought withdrawal The patient believes that thoughts are being removed from his mind by an external agency.

Thought broadcasting The patient believes that his thoughts are being 'read' by others, as if they were being broadcast.

Thought blocking Involves a sudden interruption of the train of thought, before it is completed, leaving a 'blank'. The patient suddenly stops talking and cannot recall what he has been saying or thinking.

DELUSIONS

A delusion is a fixed, false personal belief held with absolute conviction despite all evidence to the contrary. The belief is outside the person's normal culture or subculture and dominates their viewpoint and behavior.

Delusions may be described in terms of their **content** (e.g. delusions of persecution or grandeur). They can be **mood congruent** (the content of delusion is appropriate to the mood of the patient), or **mood incongruent**. Delusions are described as **systematized** if they are united by a single theme.

A **primary delusion** arises fully formed without any discernible connection with previous events (also called autochthonous delusions), e.g. "I woke up and knew that my daughter was the spawn of Satan and should die so that my son could be the new Messiah". **Secondary delusions** can be understood in terms of other psychopathology, for example hallucinations: "The neighbors must have connected all the telephones in the building; that's why I can hear them all the time".

The term delusional mood is slightly confusing in that it does not describe an abnormal belief, but refers to an ill-defined feeling that something strange and threatening is happening which may manifest as perplexity, uncertainty or anxiety. This may precede a primary delusion or a delusional perception, which involves a real perception occurring almost simultaneously with a delusional misinterpretation of that perception, e.g. "I saw the traffic lights change from red to green and knew that I was the rightful heir to the throne of England".

Overvalued ideas are unreasonable and sustained intense preoccupations maintained with a strong emotional investment but less than delusional intensity. The idea or belief held is demonstrably false and not usually held by persons from the same subculture.

Delusions may be classified in terms of their content, for example delusions of...

Persecution An outside person or force is in some way interfering with the sufferer's life or wishes them harm, e.g. "The people upstairs are watching me by using satellites and have poisoned my food".

Reference The behavior of others, objects, or broadcasts on the television and radio have a special meaning or refer directly to the person, e.g. "A parcel came from Sun Alliance and the radio said that 'the son of man is here', on a Sunday, so I am the son of God".

Control The sensation of being the passive recipient of some controlling or interfering agent that is alien and external. This agent can control thoughts, feeling and actions (passivity experiences), e.g. "I feel as if my face is being pulled upwards and something is making me laugh when I'm sad".

Grandeur Exaggerated belief of one's own power or importance, e.g. "I can lift mountains by moving my hands, I could destroy you!".

Nihilism Others, oneself, or the world does not exist or is about to cease to exist (often called Cotard's syndrome), e.g. "The inside of my tummy has rotted away. I have no bowels".

Infidelity One's partner is being unfaithful (also known as delusional jealousy or the Othello syndrome).

Doubles A person known to the patient, most frequently their spouse, has been replaced by another (also known as Capgras' syndrome or, confusingly, 'illusion' of doubles).

Infatuation A particular person is in love with the patient (also known as erotomania or de Clerambault's syndrome).

Somatic Delusional belief pertaining to part of the person's body, e.g. "My arms look like they've been melted and squashed into a mess".

THE ACUTE ILLNESS

The onset may be rapid, or slow and insidious. In the latter situation in particular, there may be a prolonged period of undiagnosed illness in which the affected person slowly becomes more withdrawn and introverted. They may develop unusual interests, particularly of a religious or philosophical kind, and drift away from family and friends. They may also begin to fail in their occupation or schoolwork. This process can take weeks to years but eventually, often with a seemingly precipitating event, the symptoms of florid illness appear.

The acute symptoms are variable but usually include delusions, hallucinations, abnormal thought processes and passivity experiences (Figures 1.11–1.16). In addition, there may be formal thought disorder, and flat or inappropriate affect. Abnormal motor signs, sometimes termed catatonic, used to be common but now are much less so in Western countries. At this stage of the illness, positive symptoms tend to dominate the clinical picture.

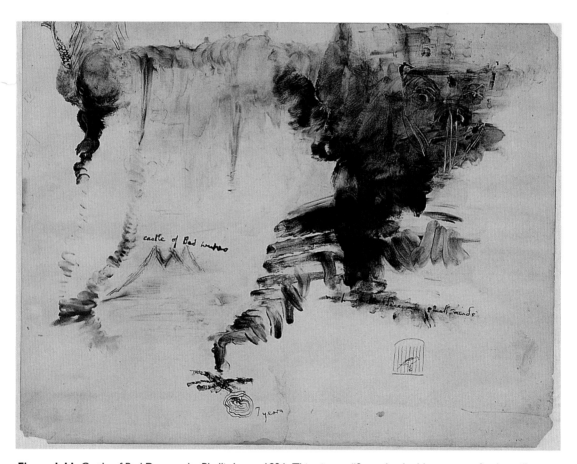

Figure 1.11 Castle of Bad Dreams, by Phyllis Jones, 1936. This picture "Served a double purpose, firstly to illustrate one of Grimm's fairytales of 'The foolish old woman' and her wishes, and secondly to symbolize her own life". It is tempting to speculate that it indicates a depressive component to her symptoms. Reproduced with kind permission of the Bethlem Royal Hospital Archives and Museum, Beckenham, Kent, UK

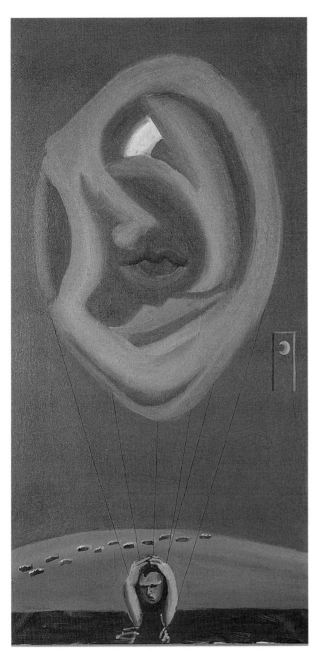

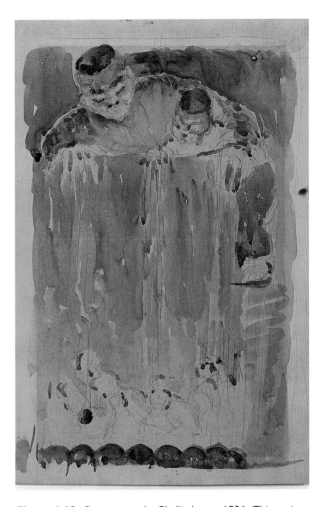

Figure 1.13 Puppeteers, by Phyllis Jones, 1936. This patient was a talented artist, who was admitted to a psychiatric hospital at the age of 22 years complaining of hearing voices, and convinced her food was being poisoned. The clinical description suggests a florid psychotic illness, of acute onset, accompanied by severe affective disturbance. Reproduced with kind permission of the Bethlem Royal Hospital Archives and Museum, Beckenham, Kent, UK

Figure 1.12 Grey self-portrait, by Bryan Charnley. This painting illustrates aspects of Charnley's psychotic symptoms, including that of hearing voices. Reproduced with kind permission of the Bethlem Royal Hospital Archives and Museum, Beckenham, Kent, UK

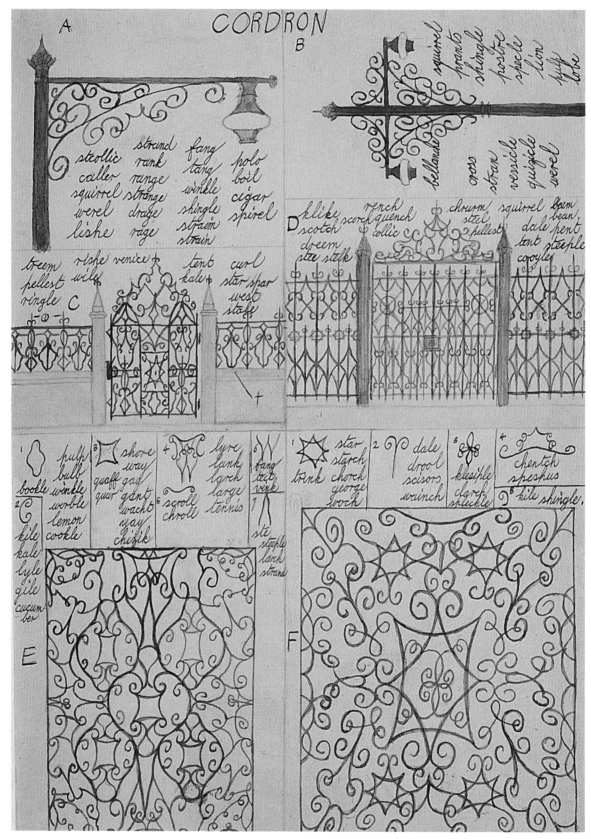

Figure 1.14 Cordron, by Gilbert Price. This patient was admitted at the age of 22 years. His extreme shyness and eccentric behavior culminated in his arrest for 'suspicious' conduct. Neologisms, elaborated into complex descriptive systems of pictures, chimneys and other objects, dominated his psychopathology. Reproduced with kind permission of the Bethlem Royal Hospital Archives and Museum, Beckenham, Kent, UK

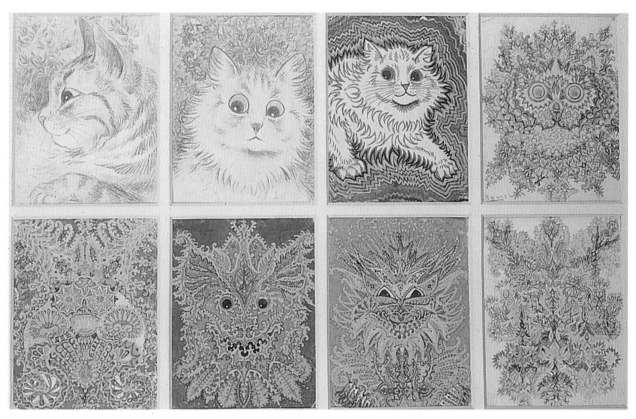

Figure 1.15 Cats, by Louis Wain (1860–1939). Wain was a British artist who became famous for his drawings of cats. He was a patient at the Bethlem Hospital in the 1920s. Paintings such as these, which are suggestive of disorganization, visual perceptual disturbances and abnormalities of affect, have been taken as illustrative of his psychological decline, although more recent scholarship suggests that they were not out of keeping with contemporary design practice. Reproduced with kind permission of the Bethlem Royal Hospital Archives and Museum, Beckenham, Kent, UK

THE CHRONIC ILLNESS

Eventually, even without treatment, the acute symptoms of schizophrenia usually resolve. Unfortunately this does not always mean that the patient will fully recover. Over 50% of patients diagnosed as suffering from schizophrenia will show evidence of a significant degree of negative symptomatology. Furthermore, in chronic schizophrenia, positive symptoms also frequently remain, although they tend not to predominate.

Negative symptoms may also be seen in the acute episode, and their onset can often precede (as one form of 'schizophrenic prodrome') the development of typical positive symptoms. Negative symptoms are multifactorial in origin. Primary negative symptoms may be difficult to distinguish from those secondary to florid positive

NEGATIVE SYMPTOMS

Poverty of speech Restriction in the amount of spontaneous speech and in the information contained in speech (alogia).

Flattening of affect Restriction in the experience and expression of emotion.

Anhedonia–asociality Inability to experience pleasure, few social contacts and social withdrawal.

Avolition-apathy Reduced drive, energy and interest.

Attentional impairment Inattentiveness at work and interview.

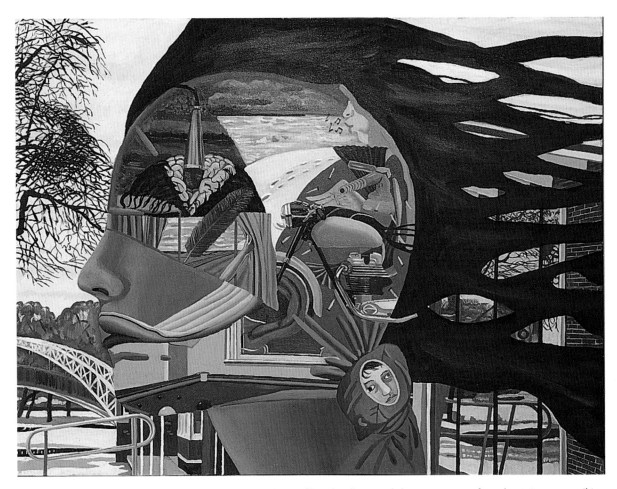

Figure 1.16 Broach shizophrene, by Bryan Charnley. Bryan Charnley illustrated the experience of psychosis in many striking artworks, including a series of self-portraits painted as he came off medication (see Figure 1.20). Reproduced with kind permission of the Bethlem Royal Hospital Archives and Museum, Beckenham, Kent, UK

psychotic symptomatology, while others may represent side-effects of antipsychotic drugs. It is often difficult to differentiate between the negative symptoms of schizophrenia and the symptoms of a depressive illness. Depression is common in schizophrenia, and often becomes evident as the acute episode resolves.

True primary negative symptoms are often described as 'deficit' symptoms. Their frequency is markedly increased in chronic schizophrenia and is related to poor prognosis, poor response to antipsychotic drugs, poor premorbid adjustment, cognitive impairment and structural brain abnormalities (sometimes called 'type 2' schizophrenia). These symptoms are not easy to treat, are often very distressing to families and carers,

and are the most important cause of long-term disability.

COURSE AND OUTCOME OF SCHIZOPHRENIA

The in-patient psychiatric population has fallen dramatically since the 1950s in Western countries, when effective antipsychotic drug treatments first became available (Figure 1.17). However, the outcome of schizophrenia, even with treatment, remains variable (Figure 1.18 and Table 1.1)[11–17].

Longitudinally, the typical course of chronic schizophrenia is described in Figure 1.19[18]. Schizophrenia also carries a high mortality. Rates of suicide in follow-up studies vary from about 2%

CHANGES IN THE IN-PATIENT PSYCHIATRIC POPULATION OF ENGLAND & WALES

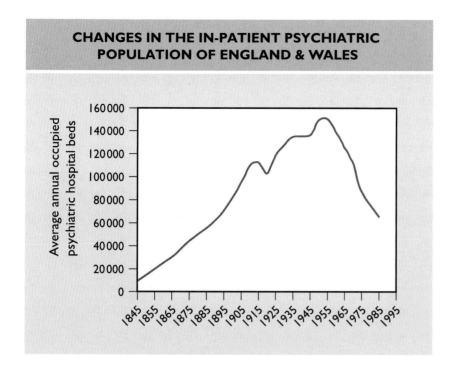

Figure 1.17 There was a steady increase in the in-patient mental hospital population in England and Wales during the hundred years from 1860. This was due to a combination of factors, including increased urbanization and changes in mental health legislation. The sharp decline in this population coincided with the introduction of effective antipsychotic medication, together with changes in health policy and legislation

FIVE-YEAR FOLLOW-UP OF 102 PATIENTS WITH SCHIZOPHRENIA

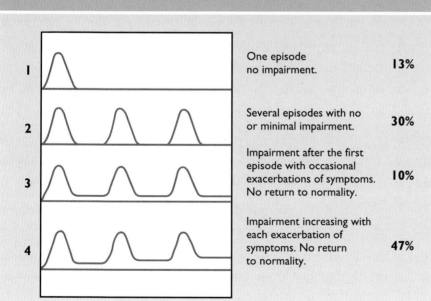

1	One episode no impairment.	13%
2	Several episodes with no or minimal impairment.	30%
3	Impairment after the first episode with occasional exacerbations of symptoms. No return to normality.	10%
4	Impairment increasing with each exacerbation of symptoms. No return to normality.	47%

Figure 1.18 Course of schizophrenia. Four typical patterns in the course of schizophrenia are described by Shepherd and colleagues[16] who followed up a cohort of patients with an operational (CATEGO-defined) diagnosis of schizophrenia who were admitted to a UK hospital over an 18-month period. Figure reproduced with permission from Shepherd M, Watt D, Falloon I, et al. The natural history of schizophrenia: a five-year follow-up study of outcome prediction in a representative sample of schizophrenics. *Psychol Med Monogr* 1989;15 (Suppl.):1–46

Table 1.1 Summary of long-term clinical outcome studies in schizophrenia.
Table reproduced with permission from Frangou S, Murray RM. *Schizophrenia*. London: Martin Dunitz, 1997

Study	Years of follow-up	Number of patients	Good clinical outcome (%)	Poor clinical outcome (%)	Social recovery (%)
Ciompi 1980[11,12]	37	289	27	42	39
Bleuler 1978[13]	23	208	20	24	51
Bland & Orne 1978[14]	14	90	26	37	65
Salokangas 1983[15]	8	161	26	24	69
Shepherd et al., 1989[16]	5	49	22	35	45

to 10% and the overall rate of suicide in schizophrenia is estimated to be in the region of 10% (Figure 1.20).

FACTORS AFFECTING PROGNOSIS

Certain clinical features are associated with a poor prognosis: early or insidious onset, male sex, negative symptoms[19,20] (Figure 1.8), lack of a prominent affective component or clear precipitants, family history of schizophrenia, poor premorbid personality, low IQ, low social class, social isolation, and significant past psychiatric history.

Several studies have demonstrated an association between longer duration of untreated illness and poorer outcome. For example, Loebel and colleagues[21] found that a longer duration of both psychotic and prodromal symptoms prior to treatment was associated with a lesser likelihood of remission. The longer the duration of pretreatment psychotic symptoms, the longer the time to remission. These data suggest that early detection and intervention in schizophrenia may be important in minimizing subsequent disability.

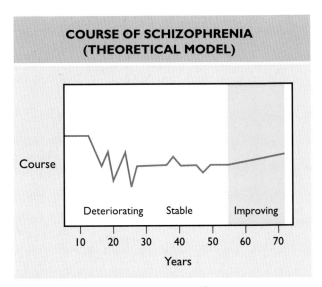

COURSE OF SCHIZOPHRENIA (THEORETICAL MODEL)

Figure 1.19 Breier and colleagues[18] among others have suggested that, despite the heterogeneity of schizophrenia, a model of a common course of illness can be derived. Based on evidence from their own studies and other long-term follow-up studies they describe an earlier deteriorating phase usually lasting some 5 years. During this time there is a deterioration from premorbid levels of functioning, often characterized by frank psychotic relapses. After this phase much less fluctuation can be expected and the illness enters a 'stabilization' or 'plateau' phase. This period may continue into the fifth decade, when there is a third 'improving' phase for many patients. Figure reproduced with permission from Breier A, Schreiber JL, Dyer J, Pickar D. National Institute of Mental Health longitudinal study of chronic schizophrenia. Prognosis and predictors of outcome. *Arch Gen Psychiatry* 1991;48:239–46

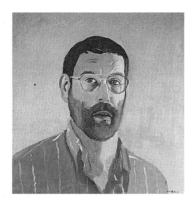

Self-portrait 11–16 April 1991

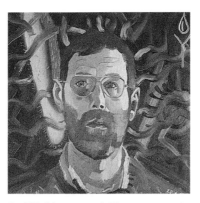

April 20: 'Very paranoid...The person upstairs is reading my mind and speaking back to me in a sort of ego crucifixion...The large rabbit ear is because I am confused and extremely sensitive to human voices, like a wild animal.'

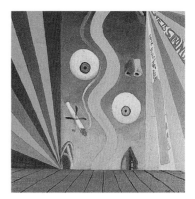

April 29: Bryan has turmoil in his mind. The features in his portrait have become fragmented. He feels lonely and exposed, as on a stage. 'A strange spiritual force is making me feel I should not smoke or I will incur a disaster.'

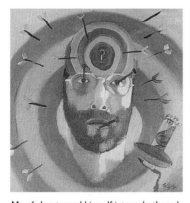

May 6: has turned himself into a dartboard. 'I feel like a target for people's cruel remarks. What is going on? I have sweet talked a girl to suicide because I had no tongue, no real tongue and could only flatter.'

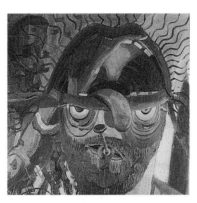

May 18: acutely disturbed. 'My mind seems to be thought-broadcasting very severely and it is beyond my will to do anything about it...I have summed this up by painting my brain as an enormous mouth.'

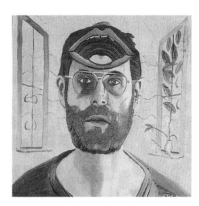

May 23: 'The blue is there because I feel depressed, through cutting back on the antidepressants...the wavy lines are because just as I feel I am safe, a voice from the street guts me emotionally by its ESP of my conditions...I am so pleased that I have been able to express such a purely mental concept as thought-broadcasting by the simple device of turning the brain into a mouth.'

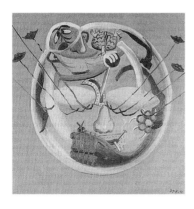

June 27 (left): This is Bryan's most complex picture. He feels he is 'closing in' on the essential image of schizophrenia. He feels transparent. 'I make crazy attempts at some sort of control over what has become an impossible situation (the man with the control stick). My brain, my ego is transfixed by nails as the Christ who could not move freely on the cross without severe pain. So I find I cannot think without feelings of pain.' The red muzzled beast symbolizes silent anger. 'My senses are being bent by fear into hallucinations.'

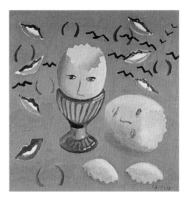

Figure 1.20 A series of self-portraits by Bryan Charnley which vividly illustrate his experiences as he came off medication. His descent into paranoia, hallucinations and depression is graphically depicted and explained with reference to his diary entries. Sadly the series ended with his death from suicide. Figures reproduced with kind permission of Mr Terence Charnley

REFERENCES

1. Haslam J. *Illustrations of Madness*. London, 1810
2. Kraepelin E. *Psychiatrie: Ein Lehruch fur Studierende und Arzte*, 5th edn. Leipzig, Germany: JA Barth, 1896
3. Kraepelin E. *Psychiatrie: Ein Lehruch fur Studierende und Arzte*, 6th edn. Leipzig, Germany: JA Barth, 1899
4. Kraepelin E. *Dementia Praecox and Paraphrenia* [1919]. Robertson GM, ed; Barclay RM, trans. New York, NY: Robert E. Kreiger, 1971
5. Bleuler E. *Dementia Praecox or the Group of Schizophrenias*. Madison, CT: International Universities Press, 1950
6. Schneider K. *Clinical Psychopathology*. Hamilton MW, trans. London, UK: Grune and Stratton, 1959
7. World Health Organization. *Report of the International Pilot Study of Schizophrenia*. Geneva: WHO, 1979
8. American Psychiatric Association. *Diagnostic and Statistical Manual, 4th Edition Revised* (DSM–IV). Washington, DC: APA, 1994
9. World Health Organisation. *The International Classification of Diseases, 10th Edition (ICD–10)*. Geneva: WHO, 1992
10. Jones P, Rodgers B, Murray R, *et al*. Child development risk factors for adult schizophrenia in the British 1946 birth cohort. *Lancet* 1994;344: 1398–1402
11. Ciompi L. Catamnestic long-term study of the course of life and aging in schizophrenia. *Schizophr Bull* 1980;6:606–18
12. Ciompi L. The natural history of schizophrenia in the long term. *Br J Psychiatry* 1980;136:413–20
13. Bleuler M. The long-term course of schizophrenic psychoses. *Psychol Med* 1974;4:244–54
14. Bland RC, Orn H. 14-year outcome in early schizophrenia. *Acta Psychiatr Scand* 1978;58:327–38
15. Salokangas RK. Prognostic implications of the sex of schizophrenic patients. *Br J Psychiatry* 1983;142: 145–51
16. Shepherd M, Watt D, Falloon I, *et al*. The natural history of schizophrenia: a five-year follow-up study of outcome prediction in a representative sample of schizophrenics. *Psychol Med Monogr* 1989;15 (Suppl.):1–46
17. Frangou S, Murray RM. *Schizophrenia*. London: Martin Dunitz, 1997
18. Breier A, Schreiber JL, Dyer J, Pickar D. National Institute of Mental Health longitudinal study of chronic schizophrenia. Prognosis and predictors of outcome. *Arch Gen Psychiatry* 1991;48:239–46
19. Johnstone EC, Frith CD, Crow TJ, *et al*. The Northwick Park 'Functional' psychoses study: diagnosis and outcome. *Psychol Med* 1992;22:331–46
20. Johnstone EC, Crow TJ, Frith CD, Owens DG. The Northwick Park 'Functional' psychoses study: diagnosis and treatment response. *Lancet* 1988; 2:119–25
21. Loebel AD, Lieberman JA, Alvir JM, *et al*. Duration of psychosis and outcome in first-episode schizophrenia. *Am J Psychiatry* 1992;149:1183–8

CHAPTER 2

Epidemiology and risk factors

The incidence of schizophrenia in industrialized countries is in the region of 10–70 new cases per 100000 population per year[1], and the lifetime risk is 0.5–1%. The geographical distribution of schizophrenia is not random: recent studies have shown that there is an increased first-onset rate in people born or brought up in inner cities (Figure 2.1)[2]. There is also a significant socioeconomic gradient, with an increased prevalence in the lower socioeconomic classes. 'Social drift', both in social class, and into deprived areas of the inner cities, may account for part of this, but specific environmental risk factors (e.g. overcrowding, drug abuse) may also be operating.

The onset of the disease is characteristically between the ages of 20 and 39 years, but may occur before puberty or be delayed until the seventh or eighth decade. The peak age of onset is 20–28 years for men and 26–32 years for women[1] (Figure 2.2). The overall sex incidence is equal if broad diagnostic criteria are used, but there is some evidence for an excess in men if more stringent diagnostic criteria, weighted towards the more severe end of the diagnostic spectrum, are

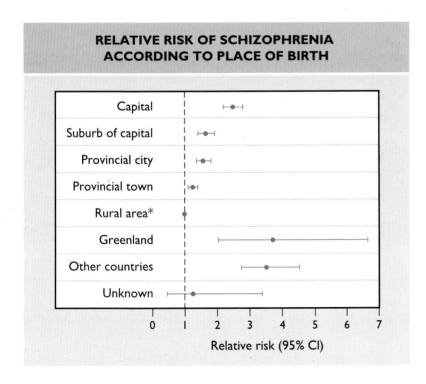

RELATIVE RISK OF SCHIZOPHRENIA ACCORDING TO PLACE OF BIRTH

Figure 2.1 Adjusted relative risk of schizophrenia in Denmark according to place of birth, with rural area used as the reference category (*). Data from reference 2

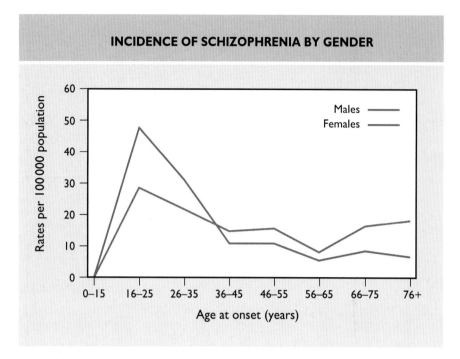

INCIDENCE OF SCHIZOPHRENIA BY GENDER

Figure 2.2 This graph shows the incidence rate per 100 000 population for broadly defined schizophrenia in an inner city area of London (Camberwell). Although the overall rate is similar in males and females, mean onset in women is slightly later. Figure reproduced with permission from Castle E, Wessely S, Der G, Murray RM. The incidence of operationally defined schizophrenia in Camberwell 1965–84. *Br J Psychiatry* 1991;159:790–4

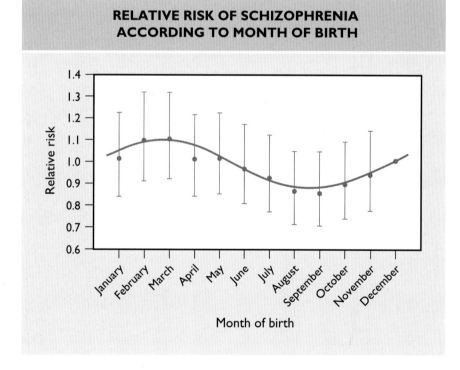

RELATIVE RISK OF SCHIZOPHRENIA ACCORDING TO MONTH OF BIRTH

Figure 2.3 This graph is based on a population cohort of 1.75 million people from the civil registration system in Denmark. The data points and vertical bars show the relative risks and 95% confidence intervals, respectively, with the month of birth analyzed as a categorical variable. The curve shows the relative risk as a fitted sine function of the month of birth (the reference category is December). Figure reproduced with permission from Mortensen PB, Pedersen CB, Westergaard T, *et al.* Effects of family history and place and season of birth on the risk of schizophrenia. *N Engl J Med* 1999;340: 603–8

applied. The prevalence of schizophrenia is considerably higher in the unmarried of both sexes. There is a small excess of patients born during the late winter and early spring months in both northern and southern hemispheres (and a less well-known decrement in late summer (Figure 2.3)[2].

People with schizophrenia have a twofold increase in age-standardized mortality rates, and are more likely to suffer from poor physical health. Much of the increased mortality occurs in the first few years after initial admission or diagnosis. Contributing factors early in the course include suicide, with later factors, such as cardiovascular disorders, due in part to the poor lifestyle of many patients, with heavy cigarette smoking and obesity being common.

THE RISK FACTOR MODEL OF SCHIZOPHRENIA

It is often said that schizophrenia is a disease of unknown etiology. This is no longer true. Schizophrenia is like other complex disorders such as ischemic heart disease, which have no single cause but are subject to a number of factors that increase the risk of the disorder. Some of the risk factors for schizophrenia are summarized in Figure 2.4. Schizophrenia, however, differs from disorders such as ischemic heart disease in that we do not understand the pathogenic mechanisms linking the risk factors to the illness, i.e. we do not understand how the causes 'cause' schizophrenia.

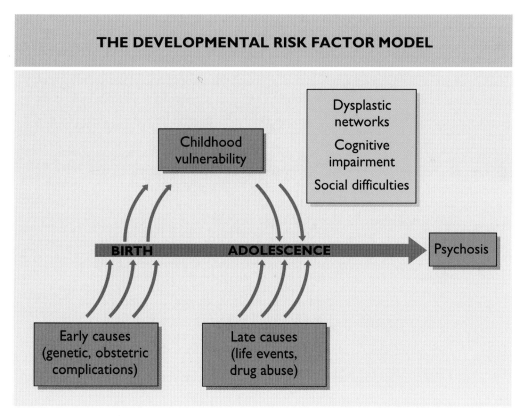

Figure 2.4 Causality over the life course. Risk factors for schizophrenia occur both early and late in the life course, and interact with each other in a complex fashion

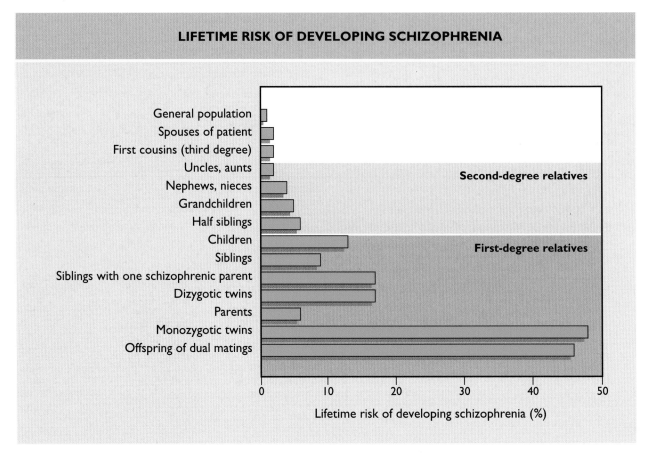

Figure 2.5 Lifetime risk of developing schizophrenia in relatives of schizophrenic individuals. Data from reference 3

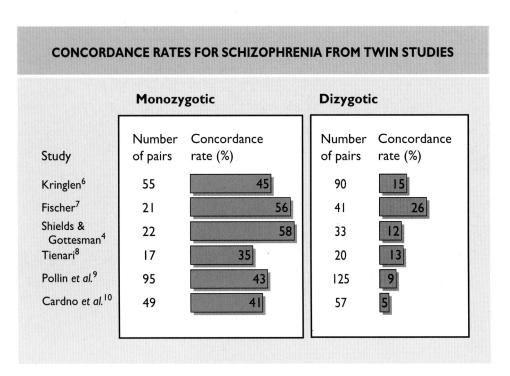

Figure 2.6 Concordance rates for schizophrenia in studies of monozygotic and dizygotic twins. The implication of the lack of 100% concordance in monozygotic twins is that there must be environmental etiological factors involved in the genesis of schizophrenia. Data from references 4–10

Relationship	Percentage schizophrenic
Parent	5.6
Sibling	10.1
Sibling and one parent affected	16.7
Children of one affected parent	12.8
Children of two affected parents	46.3
Uncles/aunts/nephews/nieces	2.8
Grandchildren	3.7
Unrelated	0.86

Table 2.1 Lifetime expectancy of broadly defined schizophrenia in the relatives of schizophrenics. Table reproduced with permission from Kendell RE, Zealley AK. *Companion to Psychiatric Studies*. Edinburgh: Churchill Livingstone, 1993

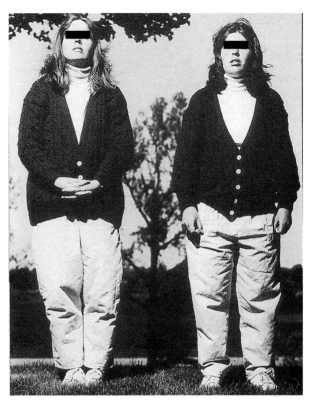

Figure 2.7 A pair of monozygotic twins discordant for schizophrenia. The twin on the right has schizophrenia

GENETICS

The most important risk factor for schizophrenia is having an affected relative (Figure 2.5 and Table 2.1)[3–5]. Twin and adoption studies have been used to show that this is consequent upon genetic transmission.

The consistently greater concordance in monozygotic (MZ) than dizygotic (DZ) twins[4–10] (Figure 2.6) has been taken to indicate a genetic effect but does not prove this beyond doubt, since MZ twins may be treated more similarly by their parents (Figure 2.7). However, adoption studies have demonstrated conclusively that liability to schizophrenia is transmitted through genes and not through some intrafamilial environmental effect (Figure 2.8)[11,12].

Various models of genetic transmission of schizophrenia have been considered but found not to fit the data. There is no evidence to support the single major locus model, which implies that a gene of major effect causes schizophrenia but has incomplete penetrance or variable expression. The polygenic model implies that there are many contributing genes, while the multifactorial model postulates that there are both genetic and environmental factors. The so-called multifactorial polygenic model involves an interaction between multiple loci and environmental factors, with schizophrenia being expressed only in individuals who exceed a certain threshold of liability.

Although the mode of transmission has not been absolutely clarified, molecular and genetic epidemiological studies concur that it is most likely to involve a number of genes of small effect interacting with environmental factors, i.e. the multifactorial polygenic model. An alternative not yet excluded is the heterogeneity model, which proposes that schizophrenia consists of several distinct conditions, each with a distinct etiology.

Molecular genetic studies have attempted to identify the particular genes that may be involved in the predisposition to schizophrenia. To date, no loci have been consistently replicated. This indicates that the susceptibility genes must each

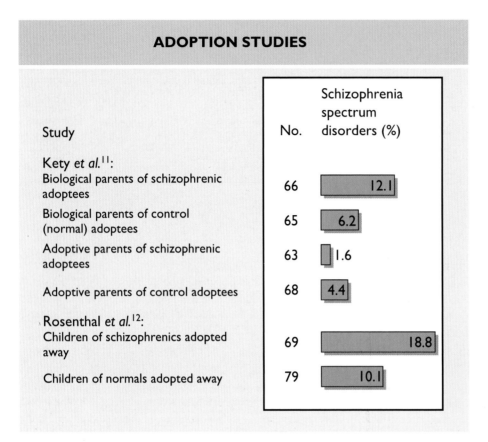

Figure 2.8 Studies of people with schizophrenia adopted away from home show conclusively that there is genetic liability to schizophrenia: there is an increase in the risk of schizophrenia associated with being a biological, but not an adoptive parent of an individual with schizophrenia. Data from references 11 and 12

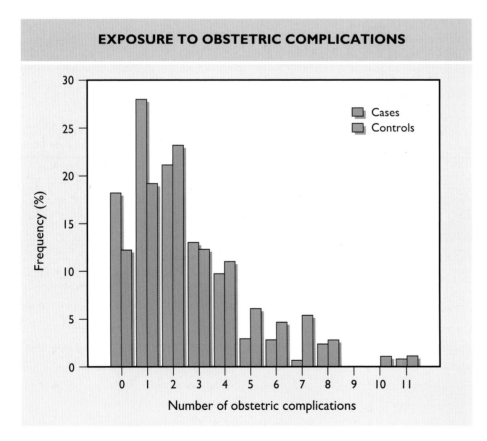

Figure 2.9 Obstetric complications are more common in people with schizophrenia compared with controls. Patients with schizophrenia are especially likely to have suffered multiple complications

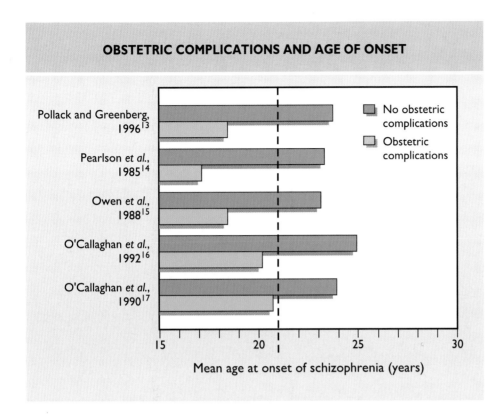

OBSTETRIC COMPLICATIONS AND AGE OF ONSET

Pollack and Greenberg, 1996[13]

Pearlson et al., 1985[14]

Owen et al., 1988[15]

O'Callaghan et al., 1992[16]

O'Callaghan et al., 1990[17]

No obstetric complications

Obstetric complications

15   20   25   30

Mean age at onset of schizophrenia (years)

Figure 2.10 Obstetric complications are a risk factor for schizophrenia in patients with a younger age of onset; they do not seem to be involved in the etiology of late-onset schizophrenia. Those patients who suffered obstetric complications showed an earlier onset than patients who did not

be of relatively small effect so as to have escaped detection. Much interest centers on so-called hotspots that may contain susceptibility genes on chromosomes 6, 8, 10, 13 and 22. There has also been interest in genes involved in the metabolism of dopamine and other catecholamines, and also in genes involved in the control of neurodevelopment.

ENVIRONMENTAL INFLUENCES

There is no doubt that there is a heritable component to the etiology of schizophrenia. It is equally clear that genetic predisposition is not the whole story. Concordance in MZ twins is only about 50%; the rest of the variance must depend on the person's environment. These are often split into early and late environmental factors (Figure 2.4).

Early environmental factors

Obstetric complications

Large population-based studies have demonstrated that obstetric complications are more common in schizophrenic populations (Figure

2.9). Meta-analyses show that exposure to obstetric complications roughly doubles the risk of later schizophrenia; however, this effect only operates for schizophrenic patients who present before the age of 25 years; obstetric complications are not involved in the etiology of late-onset schizophrenia (Figure 2.10)[13–17]. There has been a search to identify which particular obstetric complications are responsible. However, the evidence is that a range of prenatal and perinatal factors may be involved. Hypoxic ischemia has been particularly implicated; in the pre- or perinatal period this can lead to intraventricular or periventricular bleeds, resulting in ventricular enlargement; this might be one mechanism for ventriculomegaly in schizophrenia. Exocitotoxic damage associated with perinatal hypoxia may also account for some of the neurochemical abnormalities (e.g. of glutamatergic function) that are found. However, complications arising around the time of birth may reflect much earlier abnormal fetal development associated with defective genetic control of neurodevelopment and adverse environmental exposure (Figure 2.11)[18].

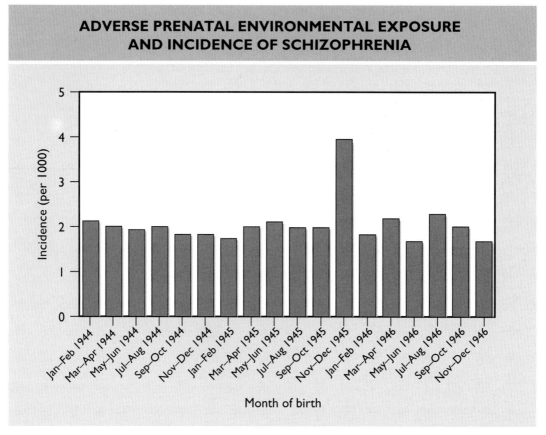

ADVERSE PRENATAL ENVIRONMENTAL EXPOSURE AND INCIDENCE OF SCHIZOPHRENIA

Figure 2.11 Exposure to nutritional deficiency during fetal development may be a risk factor for schizophrenia, as demonstrated by this study where the incidence of schizophrenia rose twofold in the group whose early fetal development occured between February and April 1945 – a period of severe famine in wartime Holland. Figure reproduced with permission from Susser E, Neugebauer R, Hoek HW, *et al*. Schizophrenia after prenatal famine: further evidence. *Arch Gen Psychiatry* 1996;53:25–31

Several studies have found men with schizophrenia to be at greater risk of obstetric complications and of preschizophrenic behavioral abnormalities, and male schizophrenics also have more marked structural brain changes. This may contribute to the fact that schizophrenia, tightly defined, is more common in men. It is also of earlier onset and greater severity, a pattern that is also seen in other neurodevelopmental disorders.

Prenatal infection

Schizophrenia is more common among those born in the late winter and early spring (Figure 2.3), so one environmental stressor potentially affecting fetal brain development that has received considerable attention is *in utero* exposure to maternal infection in the cold winter months. There is some evidence to suggest that an increase in the number of births of individuals subsequently diagnosed as schizophrenic follows influenza epidemics, although both the existence and the importance of this effect remain controversial. Exposure in later pregnancy to several other viral infections, including rubella, has also been implicated in some studies. An increase in the rate of schizophrenia has also been described among those subjected to severe malnutrition during the third trimester *in utero*[18]. Further evidence for the importance of the uterine environment in the pathogenesis of schizophrenia comes from data suggesting that preschizophrenic babies have a smaller head circumference than controls, and from studies suggesting that schizophrenic

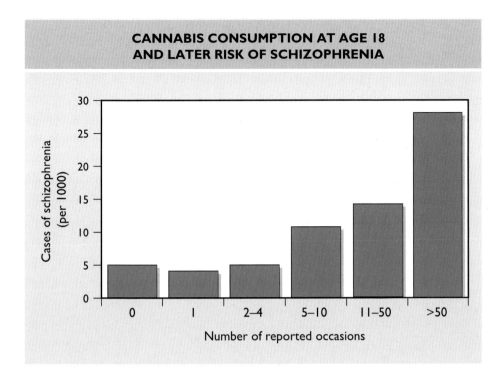

CANNABIS CONSUMPTION AT AGE 18 AND LATER RISK OF SCHIZOPHRENIA

Figure 2.12 Substance misuse can contribute to later development of schizophrenia. This study following army recruits found that those who admitted taking cannabis on more than 50 occasions had a sixfold risk of schizophrenia compared with non-users. Figure reproduced with permission from Andreasson S, Allebeck P, Engstrom A, Rydberg U. Cannabis and schizophrenia. A longitudinal study of Swedish conscripts. *Lancet* 1987;2:1483–6

patients as a group may be of lower birth weight than the general population.

Neurodevelopmental abnormality

The morphological abnormalities that have been reported in schizophrenia are consistent with a neurodevelopmental event occurring in fetal or early development. Some believe that the onset of frank psychotic symptoms reflects the delayed sequelae of an earlier developmental aberration, which is then expressed as the brain continues to develop in adolescence and adult life – sometimes termed the 'doomed from the womb' view. Delayed emergence of abnormal behavior following lesions sustained during early development is a well recognized phenomenon, and is seen, for example, in animal models where ventral hippocampal lesions, initially 'silent', are followed by hyperactivity and increased responsiveness to stressful stimuli and to dopamine blockade as the animal matures. The inherited neurodevelopmental disease metachromatic leukodystrophy is more likely to be associated with schizophreniform symptoms if the clinical onset is in adolescence. In this case, as in schizophrenia, late maturational events, such as myelination of prefrontal nerve tracts and perforant pathway, or abnormal synaptic plasticity, may reveal earlier developmental abnormalities.

Later environmental factors

Substance misuse

The relationship between substance misuse and schizophrenia is complex. Many drugs of abuse, such as ketamine, amphetamine, cocaine, and LSD, are psychotomimetic and can induce an acute schizophrenia-like psychosis. Psychoactive substance misuse both precedes and follows the onset of psychotic symptoms. Some patients state that they receive transient symptom relief and are using the drugs as a form of 'self-medication'. However, it is also clear that abuse of certain drugs can increase the risk of schizophrenia. Evidence concerning cannabis comes from the Swedish army study[19] in which army recruits were interviewed about their drug consumption and then followed-up for a decade and a half. Those who admitted taking cannabis on more than 50 occasions had a risk of later schizophrenia some six times that of non-abusers (Figure 2.12).

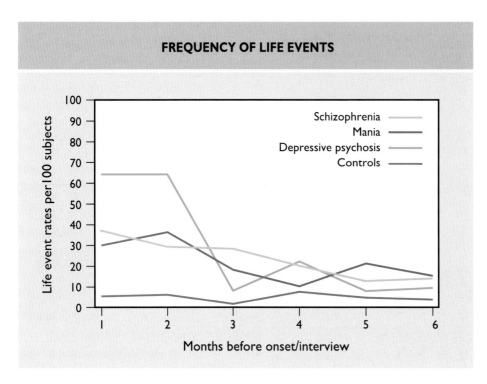

FREQUENCY OF LIFE EVENTS

Schizophrenia
Mania
Depressive psychosis
Controls

Life event rates per100 subjects

Months before onset/interview

Figure 2.13 The rate of life events is increased in schizophrenia, although the effect is not as great as in depression. Figure reproduced with permission from Bebbington P, Wilkins S, Jones P, et al. Life events and psychosis. Initial results from the Camberwell Collaborative Psychosis Study. *Br J Psychiatry* 1993;162:72–9

It is estimated that 20–50% of the population with schizophrenia in Western countries may qualify as substance abusers or 'dual-diagnosis' patients. Such patients have a higher use of services and worse outcome than patients who are not abusers; they are more likely to be hospitalized and more likely to relapse. Patients with schizophrenia seem to be more vulnerable to significant harm at relatively lower levels of substance use. As substance misuse is so prevalent in the West, this is an area where secondary prevention of relapse could be focused.

Social and psychological factors

Psychosocial factors appear to contribute to both the onset and the relapse of schizophrenia. The best documented are life events (Figure 2.13)[20]. The effect size is smaller than in depression and the time frame is somewhat shorter than in depression (where adverse life events are well recognized etiological factors), with the 3 weeks prior to onset seeming to be the most important. Unlike depression, all kinds of life events appear to be important, not just those involving loss.

Many migrant groups show an increased first-inception rate of schizophrenia compared both to the population they have left and to that which they have joined. The most striking example of this is people of African-Caribbean origin living in the UK (Figure 2.14)[1]. It seems unlikely that the factors are biological. Odegaard[21] suggested in 1933 that social isolation and alienation are the crucial factors, and most recent evidence points in this direction.

CONCLUSION

There is no single cause for schizophrenia, rather a number of risk factors (Figure 2.15) interact to propel the individual over a threshold for expression of the disease.

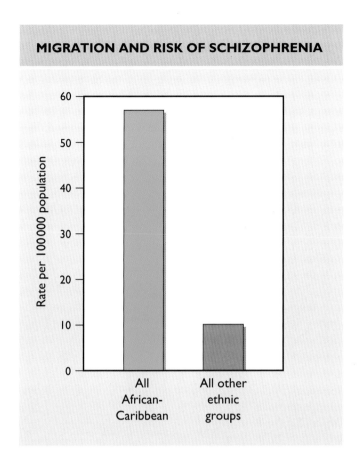

MIGRATION AND RISK OF SCHIZOPHRENIA

Figure 2.14 The differences in incidence in schizophrenia in people of African-Caribbean origin compared with those from other ethnic groups, in one study from Camberwell, South London. Figure reproduced with permission from Castle E, Wessely S, Der G, Murray RM. The incidence of operationally defined schizophrenia in Camberwell 1965–84. *Br J Psychiatry* 1991;159:790–4

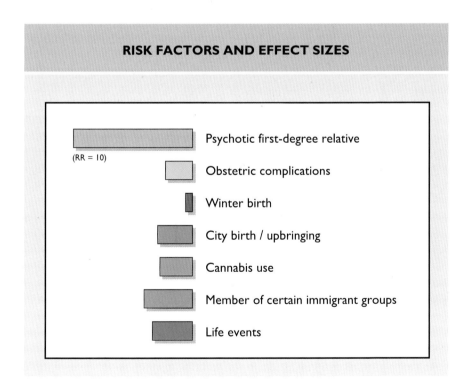

RISK FACTORS AND EFFECT SIZES

Figure 2.15 There is no single cause of schizophrenia. Instead, like other complex disorders such as coronary heart disease, a number of genetic and environmental factors interact to cause the disease

REFERENCES

1. Castle E, Wessely S, Der G, Murray RM. The incidence of operationally defined schizophrenia in Camberwell 1965–84. *Br J Psychiatry* 1991;159: 790–4

2. Mortensen PB, Pedersen CB, Westergaard T, *et al.* Effects of family history and place and season of birth on the risk of schizophrenia. *N Engl J Med* 1999;340:603–8

3. Gottesman I, Irving I. *Schizophrenia Genesis: The Origin of Madness.* New York, Oxford: WH Freeman, 1991:203

4. Shields J, Gottesman II. Obstetric complications and twin studies of schizophrenia: clarifications and affirmations. *Schizophr Bull* 1977;3:351–4

5. Kendell RE, Zealley AK. *Companion to Psychiatric Studies.* Edinburgh: Churchill Livingstone, 1993

6. Kringlen E. Twin studies in schizophrenia with special emphasis on concordance figures. *Am J Med Genet* 2000;97:4–11

7. Fischer M. Genetic and environmental factors in schizophrenia. A study of schizophrenic twins and their families. *Acta Psychiatr Scand* 1973;238 (Suppl.):9–142

8. Tienari P, Sorri A, Lahti I, *et al.* Genetic and psychosocial factors in schizophrenia: the Finnish Adoptive Family Study. *Schizophr Bull* 1987;13: 477–84

9. Pollin W, Allen MG, Hoffer A, *et al.* Psychopathology in 15,909 pairs of veteran twins: evidence for a genetic factor in the pathogenesis of schizophrenia and its relative absence in psychoneurosis. *Am J Psychiatry* 1969;126:597–610

10. Cardno AG, Marshall EJ, Coid B, *et al.* Heritability estimates for psychotic disorders: the Maudsley twin psychosis series. *Arch Gen Psychiatry* 1999;56:162–8

11. Kety SS, Rosenthal D, Wender PH, Schulsinger F, *et al.* Mental illness in the biological and adoptive families of adopted schizophrenics. *Am J Psychiatry* 1971;128:302–6

12. Rosenthal D, Wender PH, Kety SS, *et al.* The adopted-away offspring of schizophrenics. *Am J Psychiatry* 1971;128:307–11

13. Pollack M, Woerner MG, Goodman W, Greenberg IM. Childhood development patterns of hospitalized adult schizophrenic and nonschizophrenic patients and their siblings. *Am J Orthopsychiatry* 1966;36: 510–7

14. Pearlson GD, Garbacz DJ, Moberg PJ, *et al.* Symptomatic, familial, perinatal, and social correlates of computerized axial tomography (CAT) changes in schizophrenics and bipolars. *J Nerv Ment Dis* 1985; 173:42–50

15. Owen MJ, Lewis SW, Murray RM. Obstetric complications and schizophrenia: a computed tomographic study. *Psychol Med* 1988;18:331–9

16. O'Callaghan E, Gibson T, Colohan HA, *et al.* Risk of schizophrenia in adults born after obstetric complications and their association with early onset of illness: a controlled study. *Br Med J* 1992;305: 1256–9

17. O'Callaghan E, Larkin C, Kinsella A, Waddington JL. Obstetric complications, the putative familial-sporadic distinction, and tardive dyskinesia in schizophrenia. *Br J Psychiatry* 1990;157:578–84

18. Susser E, Neugebauer R, Hoek HW, *et al.* Schizophrenia after prenatal famine: further evidence. *Arch Gen Psychiatry* 1996;53:25–31

19. Andreasson S, Allebeck P, Engstrom A, Rydberg U. Cannabis and schizophrenia. A longitudinal study of Swedish conscripts. *Lancet* 1987;2:1483–6

20. Bebbington P, Wilkins S, Jones P, *et al.* Life events and psychosis. Initial results from the Camberwell Collaborative Psychosis Study. *Br J Psychiatry* 1993; 162:72–9

21. Odegaard S. Emigration and insanity. *Acta Psychiatr Scand* 1932;Suppl. 4

CHAPTER 3

Pathogenesis

Pathogenetic theories need to encompass all levels of brain structure and function, from the basic neuroanatomical level, through neurochemical, neurophysiological and neuropsychological findings, and thence through to symptoms. As yet, we have only a very partial understanding of these mechanisms.

STRUCTURAL IMAGING AND ANATOMICAL STUDIES

The core brain structural finding in schizophrenia, of lateral ventricular enlargement (Figure 3.1) is now well established, but the degree of enlargement is relatively small (Figure 3.2); about 25% on average[1]. Monozygotic twins discordant for schizophrenia can be distinguished from their co-twins on the basis of ventriculomegaly and decreased temporal cortical volume (Figure 3.3)[2]. Numerous other morphological abnormalities have been reported (Figures 3.4[3] and 3.5). People with schizophrenia appear to have very slightly smaller brains with sulcal widening and reduced cortical volume, particularly in the temporal lobes.

A number of other findings have been reported. Most of these are non-specific and tell us little about pathogenesis, but there are some clues to the processes that might be involved. Normally rare developmental abnormalities, such as agenesis of the corpus callosum (Figure 3.6), aqueduct stenosis, cavum septum pellucidum, cerebral

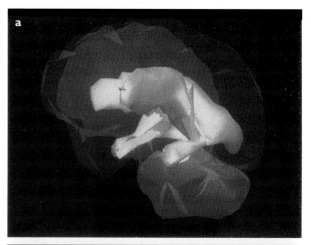
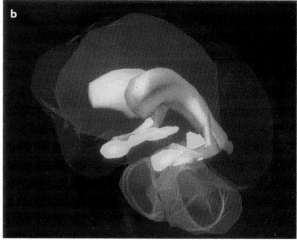

Figure 3.1 Three-dimensional reconstruction of the ventricular system in schizophrenia. Structural changes appear in the shrunken hippocampus (yellow) and enlarged fluid-filled ventricles (gray) of the brain of a patient with schizophrenia (a) compared with that of a healthy volunteer (b). Figure reproduced with kind permission of Professor Nancy C. Andreasen, University of Iowa, USA

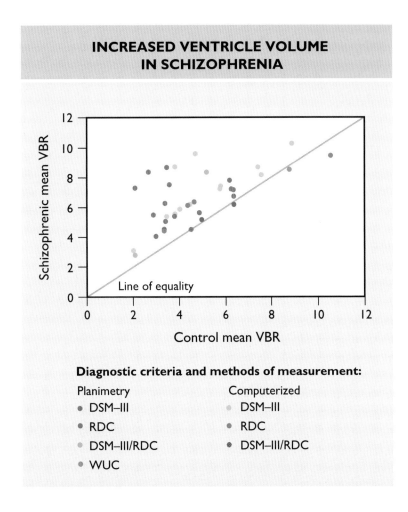

INCREASED VENTRICLE VOLUME IN SCHIZOPHRENIA

Diagnostic criteria and methods of measurement:

Planimetry
- DSM–III
- RDC
- DSM–III/RDC
- WUC

Computerized
- DSM–III
- RDC
- DSM–III/RDC

Figure 3.2 Mean ventricle : brain ratio (VBR) in controls and patients with schizophrenia from a total of 39 separate studies. The diagonal line indicates the line of equality. Thus, this figure demonstrates that no matter which diagnostic system or method of measuring brain volume is used, patients with schizophrenia do have larger ventricles than controls. Figure reproduced with permission from Van Horn JD, McManus IC. Ventricular enlargement in schizophrenia. A meta-analysis of studies of the ventricle : brain ration (VBR). *Br J Psychiatry* 1992;160:687–97

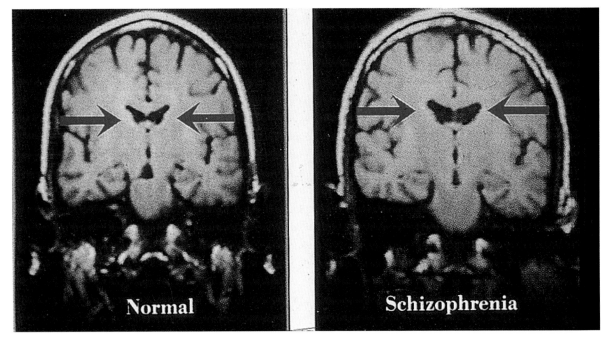

Figure 3.3 Ventricular size in monozygotic twins discordant for schizophrenia. Coronal magnetic resonance images of twins discordant for schizophrenia show lateral ventricular enlargement in the affected twin. Figure reproduced with permission from Suddath RL, Christison GW, Torrey EF, *et al*. Anatomical abnormalities in the brains of monozygotic twins discordant for schizophrenia. *N Engl J Med* 1990;322:789–4

COMPARATIVE MEAN VOLUMES OF BRAIN REGIONS IN SCHIZOPHRENIA

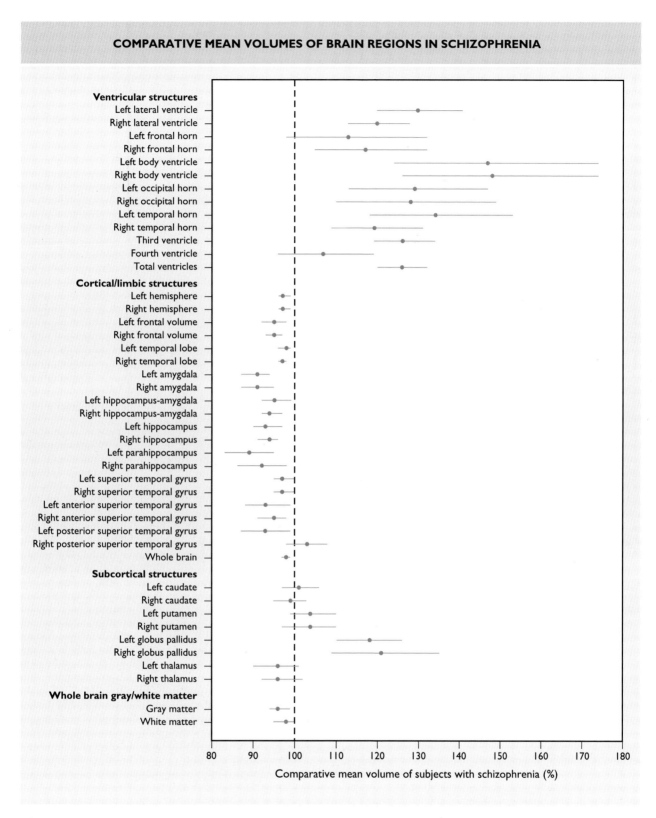

Figure 3.4 Meta-analysis of absolute regional brain volumes in schizophrenic patients and controls, from a total of 58 studies. This figure shows how the mean volumes of different brain regions from people with schizophrenia differ from those of controls. Figure reproduced with permission from Wright IC, Rabe-Hesketh S, Woodruff PW, *et al*. Meta-analysis of regional brain volumes in schizophrenia. *Am J Psychiatry* 2000;157:16–25

STRUCTURAL BRAIN ABNORMALITIES IN SCHIZOPHRENIA

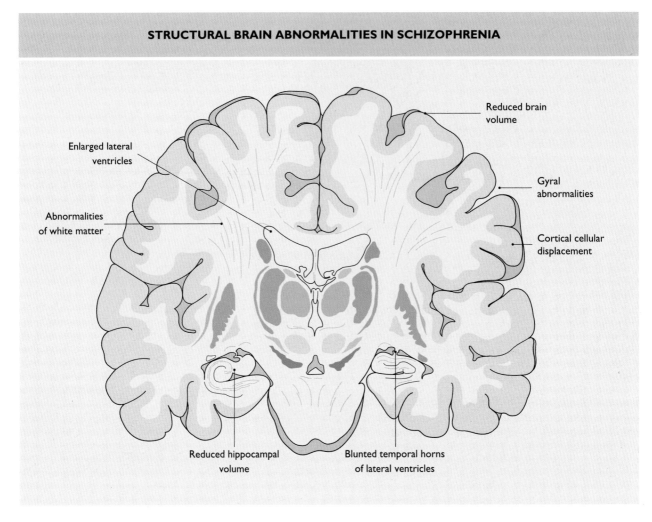

Enlarged lateral
ventricles

Abnormalities
of white matter

Reduced brain
volume

Gyral
abnormalities

Cortical cellular
displacement

Reduced hippocampal
volume

Blunted temporal horns
of lateral ventricles

Figure 3.5 Some structural brain abnormalities possibly implicated in the pathogenesis of schizophrenia. Structural abnormalities have been described in many brain areas, and at a variety of anatomical levels, from gross macroscopic changes in whole brain volume, through to subtle cellular displacement or disorganization in the cortex. Increasingly, interest has focused on the distribution of abnormalities, and their structural connectivity: thus, white matter myelination, as well as cortical abnormalities, are targets of investigation

hamartomas and arteriovenous malformations occur with increased frequency in schizophrenia.

At the cellular level, various abnormalities in cytoarchitecture have been reported in several brain regions, although not all of these findings have proved robust. However, evidence of neuronal displacement (Figure 3.7) suggests the possibility of some failure in neuronal migration, a process that occurs mainly during the second trimester of fetal development[4].

Several findings weigh against the most likely alternative of a neurodegenerative process. The balance of evidence is that most of the brain abnormalities seen in schizophrenia are present at first onset and are non-progressive. Furthermore, markers of neurodegeneration, such as proteins associated with glial response are largely absent, although there may be a small degree of periventricular gliosis. Extracerebral markers of abnormal fetal development provide indirect support for the idea that aberrant neurodevelopment is implicated in schizophrenia. Dermatoglyphic abnormalities are thought to reflect fetal maldevelopment and appear to be more common in schizophrenia (Figure 3.8). Minor physical anomalies also occur with greater frequency in

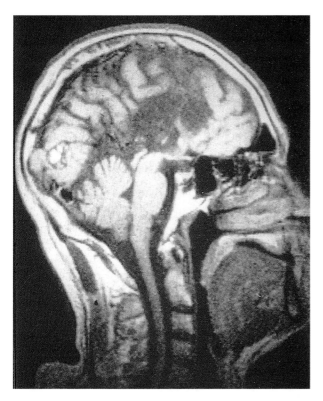

Figure 3.6 Agenesis of the corpus callosum. This midline sagittal magnetic resonance image shows an absent corpus callosum, a dramatic example of a neurodevelopmental anomaly which, while extremely rare, is thought to have an increased incidence in people with schizophrenia

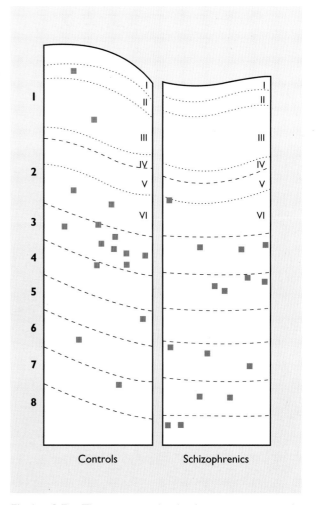

Controls   Schizophrenics

Figure 3.7 These camera lucida drawings compare the distribution of nicotinamide-adenine dinucleotide phosphate-diaphorase-stained neurons (squares) in sections through the superior frontal gyrus of a control and schizophrenic brain. There is a significant shift in the direction of the white matter in the schizophrenic brain. Numbers 1 through 8 indicate compartments of the brain; Roman numerals indicate cortical layers. Figure reproduced with permission from Akbarian S, Bunney WE, Jr, Potkin SG, *et al.* Altered distribution of nicotinamide-adenine dinucleotide phosphate-diaphorase cells in frontal lobe of schizophrenics implies disturbances of cortical development. *Arch Gen Psychiatry* 1993:50:169–77

schizophrenic patients compared with normal controls.

FUNCTIONAL BRAIN IMAGING

Functional brain imaging studies have used positron emission tomography (PET), single photon emission tomography (SPET) and, more recently, functional magnetic resonance imaging techniques (fMRI) to investigate regional cerebral blood flow (rCBF) and brain metabolism in schizophrenia (Figure 3.9)[5].

It was previously thought that a decrease in frontal blood flow and metabolism ('hypofrontality') was a constant feature of schizophrenia. However, this now appears to be a function of the cognitive load involved in the test that patients are carrying out at the time. For example, activation studies using 'frontal' tasks such as the Wisconsin

card sorting test have shown that healthy volunteers increase blood flow to the dorsolateral prefrontal cortex during the task, while this is not apparent when schizophrenic patients perform the task. Other studies using verbal fluency as an activation task have found impaired frontal blood flow in schizophrenic patients (Figure 3.10)[6]. However, there are studies on both tasks that have

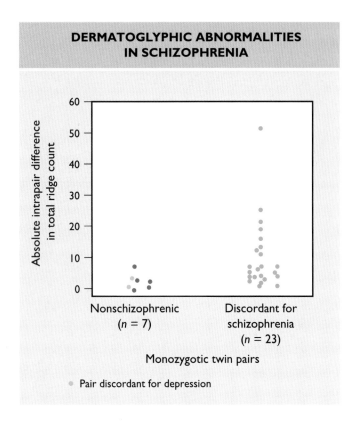

DERMATOGLYPHIC ABNORMALITIES IN SCHIZOPHRENIA

Absolute intrapair difference in total ridge count

Monozygotic twin pairs

Nonschizophrenic (n = 7)

Discordant for schizophrenia (n = 23)

- Pair discordant for depression

Figure 3.8 Structural abnormalities may be found in schizophrenia outside the CNS; other structures that develop at the same time may also be involved. In monozygotic twins there should be little or no difference between the twins in total finger ridge count. It can be seen, however, that in twin pairs where one twin suffers from schizophrenia, there is a much greater difference in total finger ridge count. This is significant because finger ridges develop in the second trimester and therefore the differences illustrated in this slide may indicate a degree of maldevelopment in affected twins

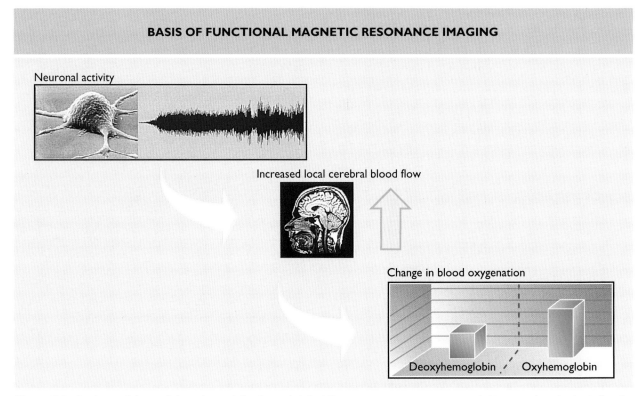

BASIS OF FUNCTIONAL MAGNETIC RESONANCE IMAGING

Neuronal activity

Increased local cerebral blood flow

Change in blood oxygenation

Deoxyhemoglobin / Oxyhemoglobin

Figure 3.9 Oxyhemoglobin and deoxyhemoglobin have slightly different magnetic properties, and this is used as the basis for the blood oxygenated level dependent (BOLD) method in functional magnetic resonance imaging (MRI). Increases in neuronal activity are accompanied by increases in regional cerebral blood flow, which exceed the increase in cerebral oxygen utilization. As a result the oxygen content of the venous blood is increased, leading to an increase in MRI signal intensity. Figure reproduced with permission from Longworth C, Honey G, Sharma T. Science, medicine, and the future. Functional magnetic resonance imaging in neuropsychiatry. *Br Med J* 1999;319:1551–4

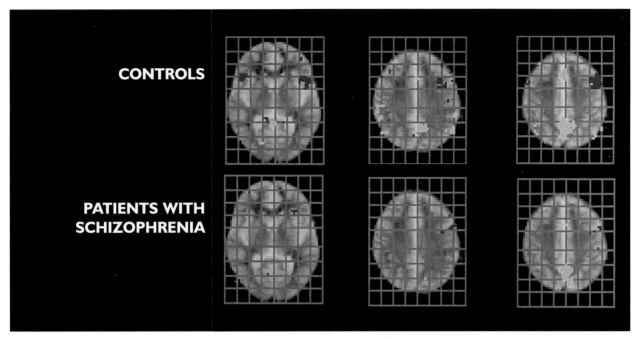

Figure 3.10 Verbal fluency and frontal lobe blood flow in schizophrenia. Comparison using functional magnetic resonance imaging between five right-handed male schizophrenic patients and five matched controls performing a covert verbal fluency task. The schizophrenic patients showed a comparatively reduced response (red) in the left dorsal prefrontal cortex and inferior frontal gyrus, and an increased response (orange) in the medial parietal cortex. Figure reproduced with permission from Curtis VA, Bullmore ET, Brammer MJ, et al. Attenuated frontal activation during a verbal fluency task in patients with schizophrenia. *Am J Psychiatry* 1998; 155:1056–63

MOTOR ACTIVATIONS AT TWO POINTS IN TIME 4–6 WEEKS APART

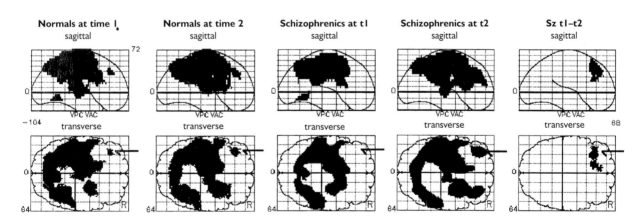

Figure 3.11 Hypofrontality in a motor activation task remitting with recovery from schizophrenic relapse. This study shows changes over time in neuronal response in a positron emission tomography study of willed action using a simple motor task. Prefrontal cortical activation not apparent at time 1 in the schizophrenic subjects (when they were acutely ill) becomes apparent at time 2, 4–6 weeks later. The figures show statistical parametric maps thresholded at $p < 0.05$, Bonferrroni corrected. Figure reproduced with permission from Spence SA, Hirsch SR, Brooks DJ, Grasby PM. Prefrontal cortex activity in people with schizophrenia and control subjects. Evidence from positron emission tomography for remission of 'hypofrontality' with recovery from acute schizophrenia. *Br J Psychiatry* 1998;172:316–23

REGIONAL CEREBRAL BLOODFLOW (rCBF)
AND SYNDROMES OF SCHIZOPHRENIA

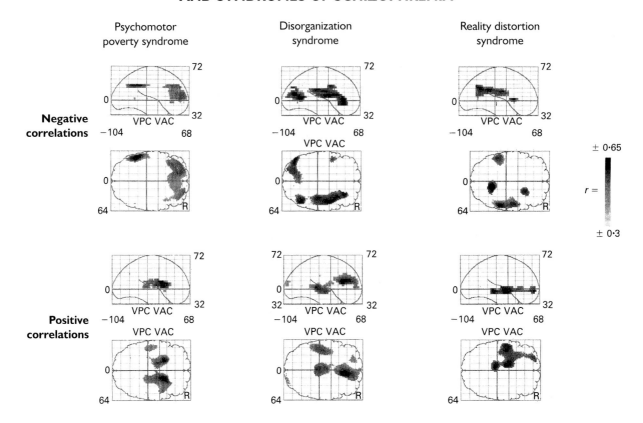

Figure 3.12 Statistical parametric maps showing pixels in which there are significant correlations between rCBF and syndrome score, for the three syndromes of psychomotor poverty, disorganization and reality distortion. Different syndromes of schizophrenia may have different patterns of aberrant rCBF. Figure reproduced with permission from Liddle PF, Friston KJ, Frith CD, *et al*. Patterns of cerebral blood flow in schizophrenia. *Br J Psychiatry* 1992;160:179–86

not shown these differences between schizophrenics and controls. Although some studies have suggested that differences in rCBF between patients and controls are persistent, others have found that they appear to be state dependent, and remit with treatment (Figure 3.11)[7].

A number of studies have attempted to correlate patterns of brain activation with specific symptoms or syndromes of schizophrenia. Liddle and colleagues[8] (Figure 3.12) investigated the three syndromes of psychomotor poverty, disorganization (i.e. inappropriate affect, speech content abnormalities), and reality distortion (i.e. delusions and hallucinations). They found that reduced rCBF in the left and medial prefrontal cortex correlated with psychomotor poverty; the severity of disorganization correlated with increased rCBF in the right medial prefrontal

cortex and decreased perfusion in Broca's area; and reality distortion correlated with increased rCBF in the left hippocampal formation. Studies of schizophrenic patients with and without auditory hallucinations have shown increased blood flow to Broca's area when patients are hearing voices. Furthermore, patients prone to auditory hallucinations show abnormal patterns of blood flow when asked to imagine hearing voices, compared with normal controls (Figure 3.13)[9], and patients with schizophrenia also appear to demonstrate abnormal patterns of temporal cortex activation in response to external speech. Abnormal patterns of blood flow also appear to be related to other specific symptoms of schizophrenia, including passivity phenomena (Figure 3.14)[10] and formal thought disorder (Figure 3.15)[11]. Interest is focusing increasingly on the

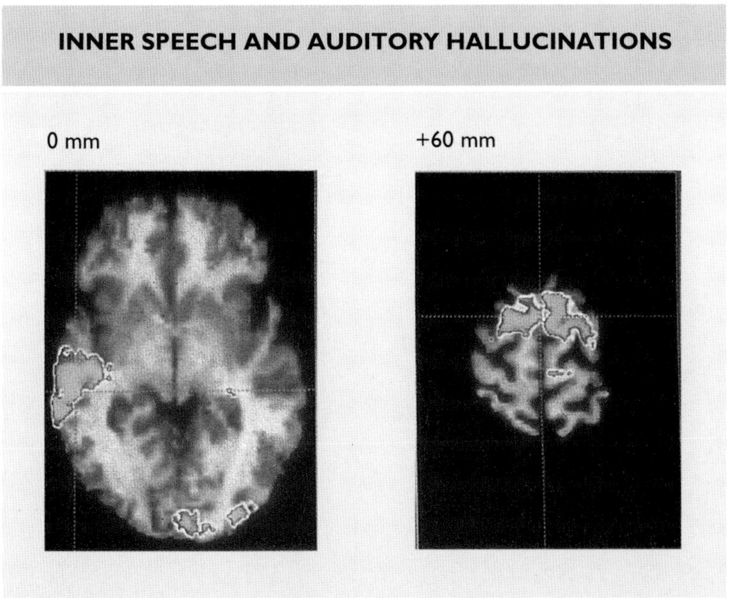

INNER SPEECH AND AUDITORY HALLUCINATIONS

0 mm

+60 mm

Figure 3.13 This study investigated the hypothesis that a predisposition to verbal hallucinations is associated with a failure to activate areas concerned with the monitoring of inner speech. Subjects, who included patients with schizophrenia both with and without a significant history of hallucinations, as well as normal controls, were asked to imagine sentences being spoken in another person's voice. The figure illustrates positron emission tomography data superimposed on a normal magnetic resonance imaging scan, and shows reduced activation in the left middle temporal gyrus and the rostral part of the supplementary motor area in hallucinators compared to non-hallucinators. Similar findings were found in the comparison between schizophrenic patients and controls. Figure reproduced with permission from McGuire PK, Silbersweig DA, Wright I. Speech: a physiological basis for auditory hallucinations. *Lancet* 1995;346:596–600

RELATIVE HYPERACTIVATION IN PATIENTS WITH PASSIVITY

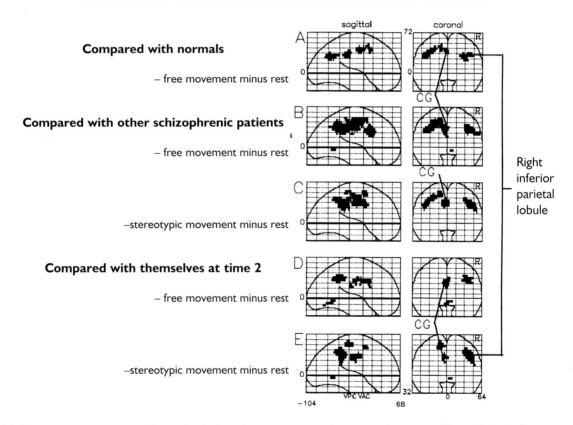

Compared with normals

– free movement minus rest

Compared with other schizophrenic patients

– free movement minus rest

C

–stereotypic movement minus rest

Compared with themselves at time 2

– free movement minus rest

E

–stereotypic movement minus rest

Right inferior parietal lobule

Figure 3.14 Positron emission tomography study of schizophrenic patients with passivity phenomena. This study looked at patients with schizophrenia who were also experiencing passivity phenomena (delusions of alien control) during a voluntary movement task. Hyperactivity is seen in these patients compared with normal controls (A), compared with other schizophrenic patients (B and C), and with themselves as their symptoms resolve (D and E). In each case, greater activation is seen in the right inferior parietal lobule (IPL), and at loci within the cingulate gyrus (CG). Figure reproduced with permission from Spence SA, Brookes DJ, Hirsch SR, *et al.* A PET study of voluntary movement in schizophrenic patients experiencing passivity phenomena (delusions of alien control). *Brain* 1997;120:1997–2011

FUNCTIONAL IMAGING OF FORMAL THOUGHT DISORDER IN SCHIZOPHRENIA

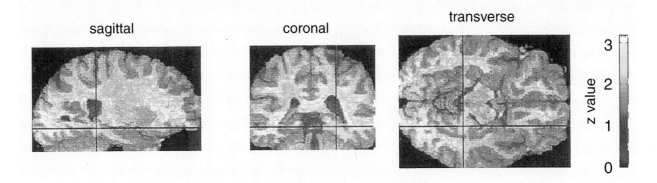

Figure 3.15 PET data have been mapped onto a normal magnetic resonance image of a brain in standard stereotactic space, sectioned to provide transverse, coronal and sagittal views. The left side of the brain is shown on the left side of the image. The images show positive correlations between the severity of positive thought disorder and regional cerebral blood flow at the junction of the left parahippocampal and fusiform gyri (marked by cross hairs), and in the anterior part of the right fusiform gyrus. Figure reproduced with permission from McGuire PK, Quested DJ, Spence SA, *et al*. Pathophysiology of 'positive' thought disorder in schizophrenia. *Br J Psychiatry* 1998;173:231–5

patterns of correlation in brain activity between different brain areas, giving rise to the concept of functional dysconnectivity, the idea that there is impaired integration of cortical activity between different areas of the brain, rather than a specific focal abnormality or group of abnormalities.

NEUROCHEMISTRY

The primary neurotransmitters implicated in the pathogenesis and treatment of schizophrenia are dopamine and serotonin. Recent theories have also implicated glutamine and γ–aminobutyric acid (GABA). The neurochemistry of schizophrenia is discussed fully in Chapter 4.

PSYCHOPHYSIOLOGY

A crucial research problem in the etiology of schizophrenia is the difficulty in confidently defining a phenotype. One of the main goals of psychophysiological research in schizophrenia has been to identify trait markers that might identify people vulnerable to developing the disorder even if they are asymptomatic.

Two promising trait markers have emerged. Eye tracking disorder, i.e. abnormalities of smooth pursuit eye movements, have been described in

people with schizophrenia and their relatives. Abnormalities in the auditory evoked potential have also been described, e.g. diminished amplitude and increased latency in the P300 response to an 'oddball' auditory stimulus, which appears to show both trait and state abnormalities (Figures 3.16 and 3.17)[12].

NEUROPSYCHOLOGY

Various theories propose mechanisms that link abnormal neuropsychology in schizophrenia to its symptoms, and the functional neuroimaging techniques described above have begun to provide an important tool in beginning to unravel these relationships. For example, schizophrenic symptoms may arise from faulty attentional processes or 'central monitoring', and, as a result, the capacity to distinguish between internal and external stimuli may be impaired (leading, for example, to the experience of hallucinations). Disorders of volition, which are clearly important at the clinical level, may also have specific neuropsychological substrates. Understanding the relationships between symptoms, cognitive function and neurochemistry has become an important new goal in researching the mechanisms of drug action.

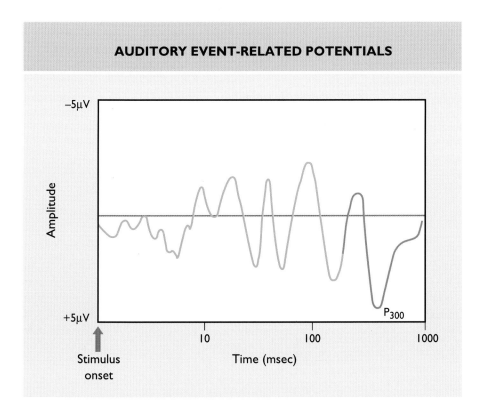

Figure 3.16 Abnormalities in evoked potentials have consistently shown abnormalities in schizophrenia. The P300 auditory event-related potential (ERP), seen here as one of several components of the auditory ERP, is seen as a response to 'oddball' or unexpected stimuli, and shows robust changes in both amplitude and latency in schizophrenic patients and their relatives.

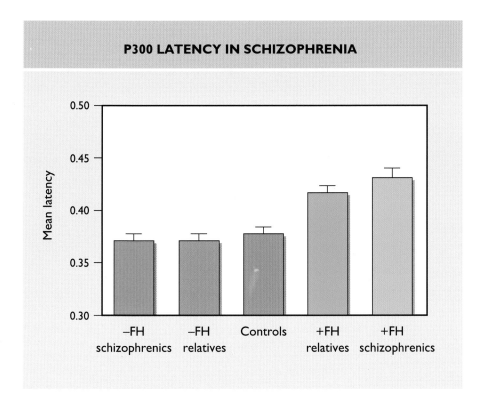

Figure 3.17 These data suggest an increased P300 latency in patients with schizophrenia and their relatives when there is a strong family history of schizophrenia (+FH), but not in sporadic cases (–FH). P300 latency may be an important trait marker for the genetic vulnerability to schizophrenia. Figure reproduced with permission from Frangou S, Sharma T, Alarcon G, et al. The Maudsley Family Study, II: Endogenous event-related potentials in familial schizophrenia. Schizophr Res 1997;23:45–53

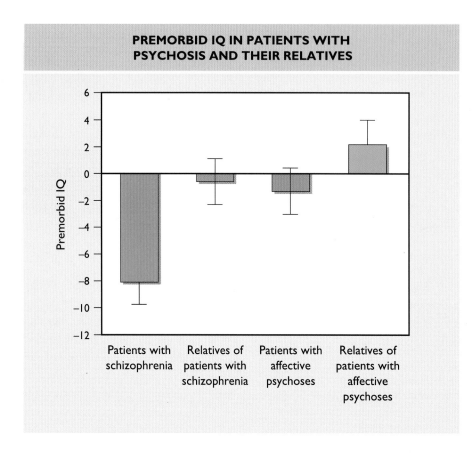

PREMORBID IQ IN PATIENTS WITH PSYCHOSIS AND THEIR RELATIVES

Figure 3.18 Deficits in premorbid IQ (as measured by the National Adult Reading Test) are seen in people with schizophrenia, but not in their first-degree relatives, or patients or relatives of patients with affective psychoses. The zero line is that of normal controls. Figure reproduced with permission from Gilvarry C, Takei N, Russell A, *et al.* Premorbid IQ in patients with functional psychosis and their first-degree relatives. *Schizophr Res* 2000;41:417–29

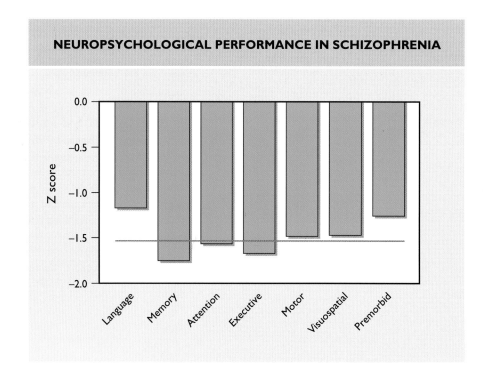

NEUROPSYCHOLOGICAL PERFORMANCE IN SCHIZOPHRENIA

Figure 3.19 Profile of neuropsychological performance of patients with schizophrenia. The deficits seen in schizophrenia are not uniform, but they encompass both executive function and memory. The zero line is the score of normal controls. Figure reproduced with permission from Bilder RM, Goldman RS, Robinson D, *et al.* Neuropsychology of first-episode schizophrenia: initial characterization and clinical correlates. *Am J Psychiatry* 2000;157: 549–59

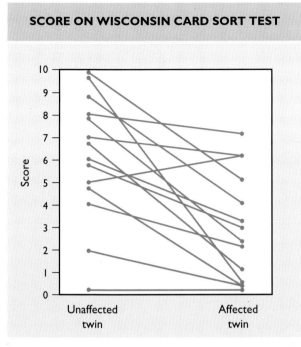

Figure 3.20 Wisconsin card sort test (WCST) in monozygotic twins discordant for schizophrenia. The WCST is a measure of executive function. In twins discordant for schizophrenia, performance on the WCST is uniformly impaired in the affected twin. Data from Goldberg TE, Torrey EF, Bigelow LB, *et al.* Genetic risk of neuropsychological impairment in schizophrenia: a study of monozygotic twins discordant and concordant for the disorder. *Schizophr Res* 1995:17:77–84

The cognitive deficits seen in schizophrenia include lower premorbid IQ (Figure 3.18)[13], as well as more circumscribed deficits, for example in memory and executive function (Figures 3.19[14] and 3.20[15]). These are almost certainly a primary feature of the disorder.

Some neuropsychological deficits are present long before the onset of schizophrenia. Two large cohort studies from the UK have supported the idea that the deficits of schizophrenia may be apparent early in life, with evidence of impaired educational test performance and avoidant social behavior (Figure 3.21)[16]. Childhood 'schizoid' personality traits may reflect deficits in cognition and in social behavior that are part of the disease process itself. Abnormalities of social behavior, movement and posture have also been reported (for example, in studies based on old home movies of affected and unaffected siblings). The antecedents of schizophrenia may therefore become identifiable long before the clinical onset of the illness.

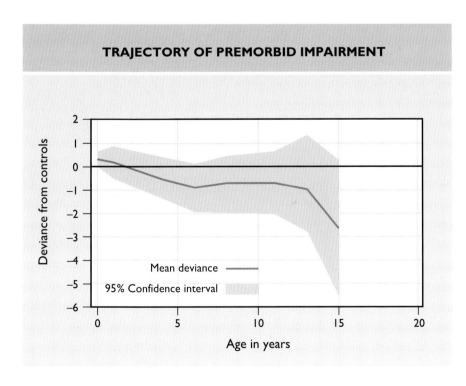

Figure 3.21 The study of large birth cohorts provides a powerful tool for investigating risk factors in schizophrenia. In the 1946 UK birth cohort[16], risk factors for later schizophrenia included problems at play, few friends, inappropriate emotional expression, anxiety, impaired intellectual function and odd movements. Figure reproduced with permission from Jones P, Rodgers B, Murray R, Marmot M. Child development risk factors for adult schizophrenia in the British 1946 birth cohort. *Lancet* 1994;344:1398–402

REFERENCES

1. Van Horn JD, McManus IC. Ventricular enlargement in schizophrenia. A meta-analysis of studies of the ventricle : brain ration (VBR). *Br J Psychiatry* 1992;160:687–97

2. Suddath RL, Christison GW, Torrey EF, *et al.* Anatomical abnormalities in the brains of monozygotic twins discordant for schizophrenia. *N Engl J Med* 1990;322:789–34

3. Wright IC, Rabe-Hesketh S, Woodruff PW, *et al.* Meta-analysis of regional brain volumes in schizophrenia. *Am J Psychiatry* 2000;157:16–25

4. Akbarian S, Bunney WE, Jr, Potkin SG, *et al.* Altered distribution of nicotinamide-adenine dinucleotide phosphate-diaphorase cells in frontal lobe of schizophrenics implies disturbances of cortical development. *Arch Gen Psychiatry* 1993:50:169–77

5. Longworth C, Honey G, Sharma T. Science, medicine, and the future. Functional magnetic resonance imaging in neuropsychiatry. *Br Med J* 1999;319:1551–4

6. Curtis VA, Bullmore ET, Brammer MJ, *et al.* Attenuated frontal activation during a verbal fluency task in patients with schizophrenia. *Am J Psychiatry* 1998;155:1056–63

7. Spence SA, Hirsch SR, Brooks DJ, Grasby PM. Prefrontal cortext activity in people with schizophrenia and control subjects. Evidence from positron emission tomography for remission of 'hypofrontality' with recovery from acute schizophrenia. *Br J Psychiatry* 1998;172:316–23

8. Liddle PF, Friston KJ, Frith CD, *et al.* Patterns of cerebral blood flow in schizophrenia. *Br J Psychiatry* 1992;160:179–86

9. McGuire PK, Silbersweig DA, Wright I. Speech: a physiological basis for auditory hallucinations. *Lancet* 1995;346:596–600

10. Spence SA, Brookes DJ, Hirsch SR, *et al.* A PET study of voluntary movement in schizophrenic patients experiencing passivity phenomena (delusions of alien control). *Brain* 1997;120:1997–2011

11. McGuire PK, Quested DJ, Spence SA, *et al.* Pathophysiology of 'positive' thought disorder in schizophrenia. *Br J Psychiatry* 1998;173:231–5J

12. Frangou S, Sharma T, Alarcon G, *et al.* The Maudsley Family Study, II: Endogenous event-related potentials in familial schizophrenia. *Schizophr Res* 1997; 23:45–53

13. Gilvarry C, Takei N, Russell A, *et al.* Premorbid IQ in patients with functional psychosis and their first-degree relatives. *Schizophr Res* 2000;41:417–29

14. Bilder RM, Goldman RS, Robinson D, *et al.* Neuropsychology of first-episode schizophrenia: initial characterization and clinical correlates. *Am J Psychiatry* 2000;157:549–59

15. Goldberg TE, Torrey EF, Bigelow LB, *et al.* Genetic risk of neuropsychological impairment in schizophrenia: a study of monozygotic twins discordant and concordant for the disorder. *Schizophr Res* 1995: 17:77–84

16. Jones P, Rodgers B, Murray R, Marmot M. Child development risk factors for adult schizophrenia in the British 1946 birth cohort. *Lancet* 1994;344: 1398–402

CHAPTER 4

Neurochemistry and pharmacotherapy

INTRODUCTION

The discovery of the antipsychotic effects of chlorpromazine in the early 1950s heralded an era of effective pharmacological treatment for schizophrenia. Since the initial 1952 report of reduction in agitation, aggression and delusional states in schizophrenic patients, a wealth of placebo-controlled trials have established the efficacy of typical antipsychotic (neuroleptic) medication for acute schizophrenia, and for maintenance in chronic schizophrenia.

Antipsychotics are therefore the mainstay of treatment in schizophrenia and knowledge of the chemistry and pharmacology of these medications has led to a greater understanding of the neurochemical basis of schizophrenia.

Table 4.1 The classification of antipsychotic drugs. The relevance of classifying antipsychotics according to their chemical class is seen when switching antipsychotics. Patients who do not respond to a medication coming from a particular chemical class should be switched to a medication of a different chemical class. The emphasis is now changing to pharmacological rather than chemical classes, as all of the newer medications belong to different chemical classes, but some share similar pharmacological properties

Type	Class	Examples
Typical antipsychotics	phenothiazines	chloropromazine, thioridazine trifluoperazine, fluphenazine
	butyrophenones	haloperidol, droperidol
	thioxanthenes	flupenthixol, zuclopenthixol
	diphenylbutylpiperidines	pimozide, fluspiraline
Atypical antipsychotics	dibenzodiazepines	clozapine
	benzixasoles	risperidone, iloperidone
	thienobenzodiazepines	olanzapine
	dibenzothiazepines	quetiapine
	imidazolidinones	sertindole
	benzothiazolylpiperazines	ziprasidone
	substituted benzamides	amisulpride, sulpiride (NB. sulpiride is considered by some to be a typical antipsychotic)
	quinolinones	aripiprazole

AFFINITY FOR DOPAMINE RECEPTORS AND CLINICAL POTENCY

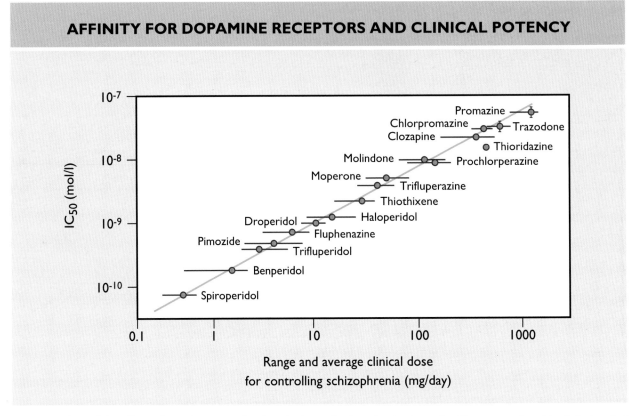

Figure 4.1 Plot of the affinity of a wide variety of antipsychotic medications for the dopamine D_2 receptor (y-axis), plotted against the average clinical daily dose used for controlling schizophrenia (x-axis), an estimate of clinical potency. As can be seen, there is a direct relationship between these two indices. This replicated finding contributed to the use of high-dose antipsychotics on the assumption that giving higher doses would make an antipsychotic more potent by 'blocking' more receptors

CLASSIFICATION OF ANTIPSYCHOTICS

Antipsychotic drugs are not a homogeneous group, and there are various classes. The phenothiazines include chlorpromazine, trifluoperazine and fluphenazine. Other classes include the thioxanthenes (e.g. flupenthixol and zuclopenthixol) and the butyrophenones (e.g. haloperidol) (Table 4.1). The newer 'atypical' antipsychotics are mostly in different chemical classes, although they may share pharmacological characteristics.

NEUROCHEMISTRY OF SCHIZOPHRENIA AND MECHANISMS OF ACTION OF ANTIPSYCHOTICS

Dopamine

The observation from the early use of chlorpromazine that clinical improvement was often accompanied by a parkinsonism-like syndrome led to a focus on dopaminergic mechanisms of action for antipsychotics. In 1963 Carlsson and Lindqvist[1] reported that antipsychotics increased turnover of brain dopamine, and suggested that this was in response to a functional 'blockade' of the dopaminergic system. Creese and colleagues[2] demonstrated that the affinity of a wide range of antipsychotics to dopamine D_2 receptors was proportionate to their clinical potency (Figure 4.1). Further evidence for the dopamine hypothesis is that amphetamines, which increase dopamine release, can induce a paranoid psychosis and exacerbate schizophrenia and that disulfiram inhibits dopamine hydroxylase and exacerbates schizophrenia[3,4].

Initial positron emission tomography (PET) studies of D_2 receptor densities in drug-naive and drug-free patients with schizophrenia, using different tracers, were equivocal, with one group showing a marked increase in receptor density and

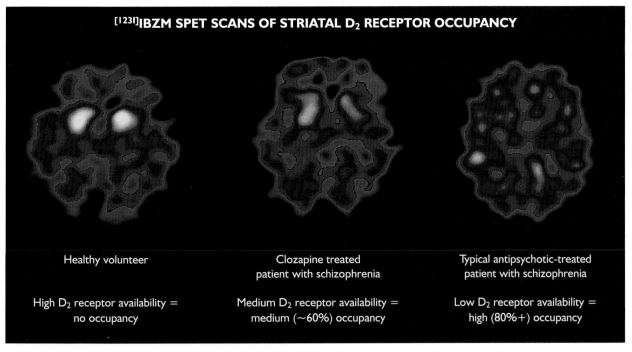

Figure 4.2 Three single photon emission tomography (SPET), scans of striatal D_2 and D_2-like receptor availability at the level of the basal ganglia. In the scan on the left from a healthy volunteer there is no receptor occupancy and therefore 100% receptor availability for the binding of the D_2 receptor tracer [123I]IBZM. The scan on the right is from a patient with schizophrenia receiving a typical antipsychotic. The bright areas from the left hand scan indicating high receptor density are not evident on the right-hand scan as the antipsychotic is occupying the majority of the receptors and preventing the tracer from binding. Unfortunately despite this high level of occupancy this patient has failed to respond to treatment. The central scan is from a patient receiving clozapine, although the striatum are not as 'bright' as in the healthy volunteer they are visible. This scan indicates intermediate occupancy of the receptors by clozapine. Importantly the patient with the intermediate occupancy has responded to treatment. Studies such as this one, when performed in larger groups, indicate that the simple dopamine hypothesis suggested by the data in Figure 4.1 needed refining. Figure reproduced with permission from Pilowsky LS, Costa DC, Ell PJ, et al. Clozapine, single photon emission tomography, and the D_2 dopamine receptor blockade hypothesis of schizophrenia. *Lancet* 1992;340:199–202

another showing no change[5]. Although the majority of subsequent studies with PET or SPET have found no significant difference in striatal D_2 receptor density between controls and patients with schizophrenia, in a recent meta-analysis of studies carried out between 1986 and 1997, a small but significant elevation of D_2 receptors was noted in patients with schizophrenia[5]. However, the variability of D_2 receptor density is high both in controls and patients with schizophrenia, and it has been argued that the small magnitude of the effect (approximately a 12% increase), and the possibility that any change reflects alteration in the baseline synaptic dopamine, means that there are no real functional differences in the density of striatal D_2 receptors in schizophrenia (reviewed in reference 5).

Despite these equivocal findings in drug-naive patients, emission tomography has reinforced the accepted theory that antipsychotic efficacy is related to D_2, with 65% blockade a putative threshold for antipsychotic response[6]. Nonetheless, the situation appears very complex in that non-responders to antipsychotics still show high levels of striatal D_2 blockade[7,8]. Furthermore, the highly effective atypical antipsychotic clozapine produces far less striatal D_2 blockade than typical antipsychotics[7–9], often below the putative 65% threshold (Figure 4.2). These findings have yet to be fully explained.

Extrapyramidal side-effects (EPS) have also been studied and a threshold of 80% D_2 occupancy has been repeatedly shown to be necessary to produce EPS[6] (Figure 4.3). It may be that high levels of 5-HT_{2A} receptor blockade, as seen with

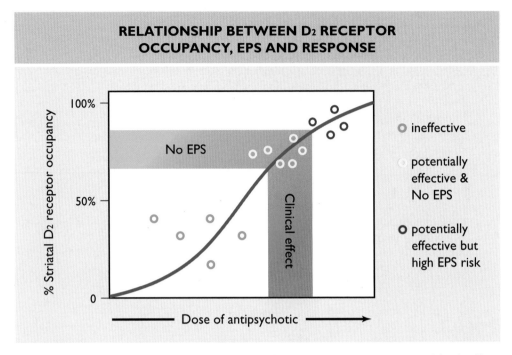

Figure 4.3 Illustration of the relationship between clinical effectiveness, extrapyramidal side-effects (EPS) and D$_2$ receptor occupancy. With the exception of clozapine-induced D$_2$ occupancy, below 60% striatal D$_2$ occupancy produced by an antipsychotic medication is likely to be associated with treatment non-response, whilst occupancies above 80% are likely to be associated with a high risk of EPS. Once a patient is receiving a dose of an antipsychotic likely to be producing an occupancy between 60% and 80% there is little to be gained, in terms of treatment response, by increasing the dose of the antipsychotic further as the patient will almost certainly develop EPS. Figure after references 6, 7 and 51

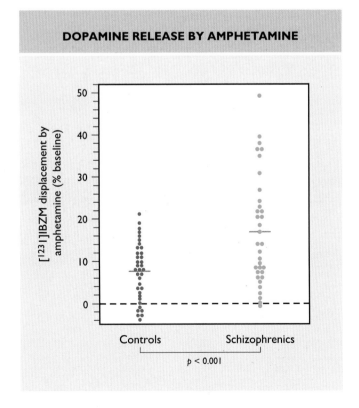

Figure 4.4 The effect of amphetamine (0.3 mg/kg) on [123I]IBZM binding in healthy control subjects and untreated patients with schizophrenia. [123I]IBZM is a tracer for D$_2$ receptors which allows *in vivo* measurement of D$_2$ receptor availability (or binding potential) in humans using single photon emission tomography (SPET). The y-axis shows the percentage decrease in [123I]IBZM binding potential induced by amphetamine, which is a measure of the increased occupancy of D$_2$ receptors by dopamine following the challenge. Thus, these results indicate that, when challenged with amphetamine, patients with schizophrenia release more dopamine than do healthy controls. Figure reproduced with permission from Laruelle M, Abi-Dargham A, Gil R, *et al.* Increased dopamine transmission in schizophrenia: relationship to illness phases [Review]. *Biol Psychiatry* 1999; 46:56–72

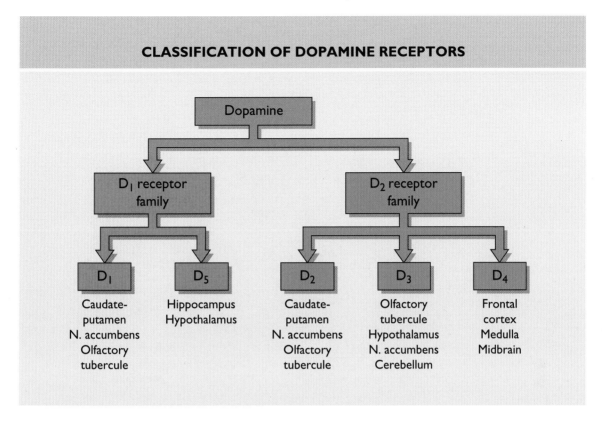

CLASSIFICATION OF DOPAMINE RECEPTORS

Figure 4.5 There are currently five types of dopamine receptor identified in the human nervous system, D_1 to D_5. D_1 and D_5 receptors are similar in that they both stimulate the formation of cAMP by activation of a stimulatory G-coupled protein. D_1 and D_5 are therefore known as D_1-like receptors. D_2 to D_4 receptors activate an inhibitory G-protein, thereby inhibiting the formation of cAMP. They are collectively known as D_2-like receptors. D_2 receptors are more ubiquitous than D_3 or D_4 receptors. D_3 receptors are differentially situated in the nucleus accumbens (one of the septal nuclei in the limbic system) and D_4 receptors are especially concentrated in the frontal cortex

most of the newer antipsychotics, may be protective against EPS by altering this threshold (reviewed in reference 10).

Recent neurochemical imaging studies have indicated that people with schizophrenia have an increased sensitivity of their dopaminergic neurones to amphetamine challenge[11] (Figure 4.4). Thus, it may be that in response to 'stress' such people will over-release dopamine and this may drive psychosis.

There are currently five types of dopamine receptors identified in the human nervous system: D_1 to D_5. D_1 and D_5 receptors are similar in that they both stimulate the formation of cAMP by activation of a stimulatory G-coupled protein. D_2 to D_4 receptors act by activating an inhibitory G-protein, thereby inhibiting the formation of cAMP. D_2 receptors are more ubiquitous than D_3 or D_4 receptors. D_3 receptors are differentially situated in the nucleus accumbens (one of the septal nuclei in the limbic system) and D_4 receptors are especially concentrated in the frontal cortex (Figure 4.5). There are a number of different dopaminergic pathways or tracts (Figure 4.6). The nigrostriatal tract projects from the substantia nigra in the midbrain to the corpus striatum. This tract primarily has a role in motor control, although the ventral striatum has a role in reward- and goal-directed behaviors. Degeneration of the cells in the substantia nigra leads to idiopathic Parkinson's disease, and it is by blocking the dopamine receptor at the termination of this pathway that the parkinsonian side-effects of classical antipsychotics arise. The mesolimbic/mesocortical tract has its cell bodies in the ventral tegmental area adjacent to the substantia nigra. This tract projects to the limbic system and neocortex in addition to the striatum. This

THE DOPAMINERGIC PATHWAYS

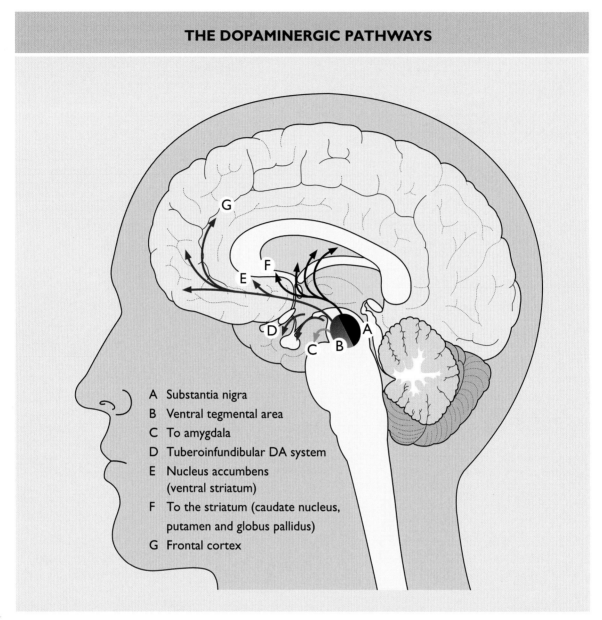

A Substantia nigra
B Ventral tegmental area
C To amygdala
D Tuberoinfundibular DA system
E Nucleus accumbens
   (ventral striatum)
F To the striatum (caudate nucleus,
   putamen and globus pallidus)
G Frontal cortex

Figure 4.6 Representation of the primary dopamine-containing tracts in the human brain. The nigrostriatal tract is primarily involved in motor control, but also in reward- and goal-directed behavior. Blockade of D_2 receptors here produces some of the antipsychotic effects of antipsychotics, but high levels of blockade (> 80%) produce parkinsonian side-effects. Blockade of D_2 receptors in the tuberoinfundibular pathway increases plasma prolactin. It is thought that it is the blockade of D_2 and D_2-like receptors in the mesolimbic and mesocortical tracts that underlies the primary antipsychotic effects of all currently available antipsychotics

dopaminergic innervation supplies fibers to the medial surface of the frontal lobes and to the parahippocampus and cingulate cortex, the latter two being part of the limbic system. Because of this anatomic representation it is thought that this tract is where antipsychotic medication exerts its beneficial effect. The third major pathway is termed the tuberoinfundibular tract. The cell bodies for this tract reside in the arcuate nucleus and periventricular area of the hypothalamus. They project to the infundibulum and the anterior pituitary. Dopamine acts within this tract to inhibit the release of prolactin. The blockade of these receptors by antipsychotics removes the inhibitory drive from prolactin release and leads to prolactinemia.

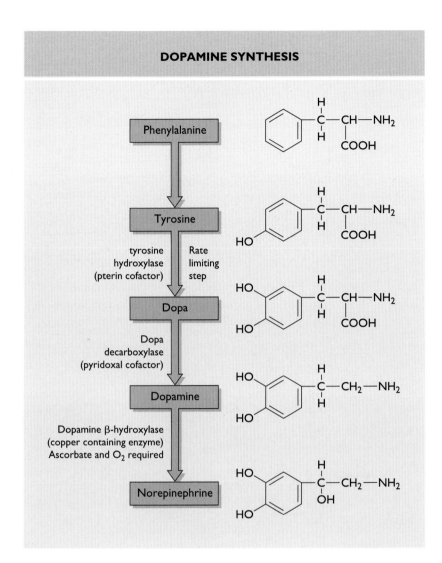

DOPAMINE SYNTHESIS

Figure 4.7 Dopamine is synthesized in a common pathway with norepinephrine. In the pathway shown, tyrosine hydroxylase is the rate-limiting enzyme. Dopamine β-hydroxylase is only found in noradrenaline neurons in the CNS

Figure 4.8 Dopamine is metabolized by two enzymes. One, monoamine oxidase type B (MAO-B), is intraneuronal, and the other, catechol-O-methyl transferase (COMT), is extraneuronal. The primary metabolite of dopamine is homovanillic acid

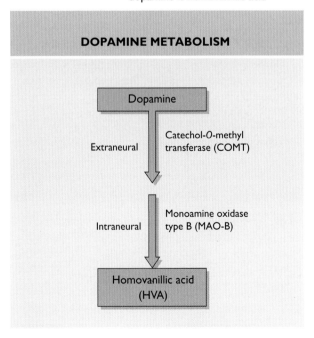

DOPAMINE METABOLISM

Dopamine is synthesized as part of the common pathway for catecholamines (Figure 4.7). Dopamine is metabolized by two enzymes; one, monoamine oxidase type B (MAO-B), is intraneuronal, and the other, catechol-O-methyl transferase (COMT), is extraneuronal. The primary metabolite of dopamine is homovanillic acid (HVA; Figure 4.8).

Serotonin

The serotonergic hypothesis of schizophrenia predates the dopaminergic hypothesis and stems from the finding by Woolley and Shaw in 1954[12] that the hallucinogen LSD acted via serotonin.

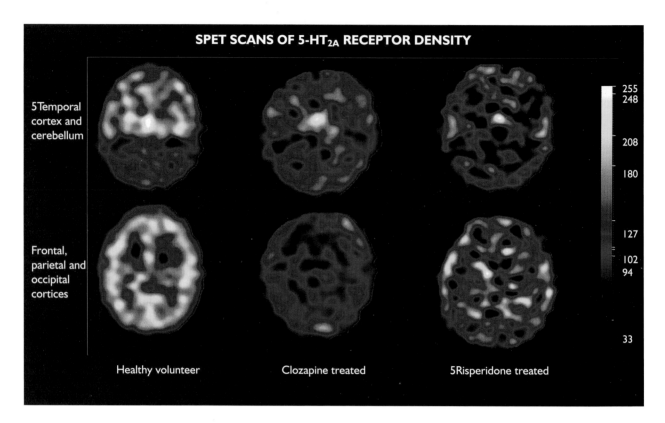

SPET SCANS OF 5-HT₂ₐ RECEPTOR DENSITY

5 Temporal cortex and cerebellum

Frontal, parietal and occipital cortices

Healthy volunteer   Clozapine treated   5 Risperidone treated

255
248

208

180

127

102
94

33

Figure 4.9 Single photon emission tomography (SPET) scans of 5-HT₂ₐ receptor density in a healthy volunteer and two patients with schizophrenia receiving a therapeutic dose of either clozapine (450 mg/day) or risperidone (6 mg/day). In the slice at the level of the frontal, parietal and occipital cortices from the healthy volunteer the ubiquitous distribution of 5-HT₂ₐ receptors in the cortical gray matter can be seen. This binding of the tracer is absent from the equivalent slices from the medicated patients. This indicates that both clozapine and risperidone are producing very high or 'saturation' levels of 5-HT₂ₐ receptor blockade. This high level of blockade may confer some protection against the development of EPS and may be one of the mechanisms of antipsychotic 'atypicality'. Figure reproduced with permission from Travis MJ, Busatto GF, Pilowsky LS, et al. 5-HT₂ₐ receptor blockade in patients with schizophrenia treated with risperidone or clozapine. A SPET study using the novel 5-HT₂ₐ ligand 123I-5-I-R-91150. Br J Psychiatry 1998;173:236–41

There is a neuroanatomical and functional interaction of 5-HT and dopaminergic systems such that blocking 5-HT₂ₐ receptors enhances dopaminergic transmission. The newer atypical antipsychotics, in contrast with the typical antipsychotics, all have a higher affinity for the 5-HT₂ₐ receptor than for the D₂ receptor. In terms of treatment response, there is a correlation of serotonergic neuroendocrine responses with symptomatic improvement on clozapine and preliminary data suggesting that allelic variations in the 5-HT₂ₐ receptor gene vary with, and may predict, treatment response[10].

PET studies of 5-HT₂ₐ receptor density in drug-naive patients with schizophrenia have failed to show any difference in comparison with matched healthy controls[13,14]. Previous studies with PET and SPET have indicated that the 'atypical' and newer antipsychotic medications like clozapine, risperidone, olanzapine and sertindole all lead to almost complete occupancy of cortical 5-HT₂ₐ receptors at clinically relevant doses[15-17] (Figure 4.9) Full characterization of the effects of the older typical antipsychotics on 5-HT₂ₐ receptors remains to be completed, however, preliminary data indicates that broad-spectrum typical antipsychotics such as phenothiazines and thioxanthines also lead to a significant occupancy (or reduction in receptor availability) of cortical 5-HT₂ₐ receptors, but the level of occupancy is still significantly lower than that seen with the newer medications[18].

SEROTONINERGIC PATHWAYS

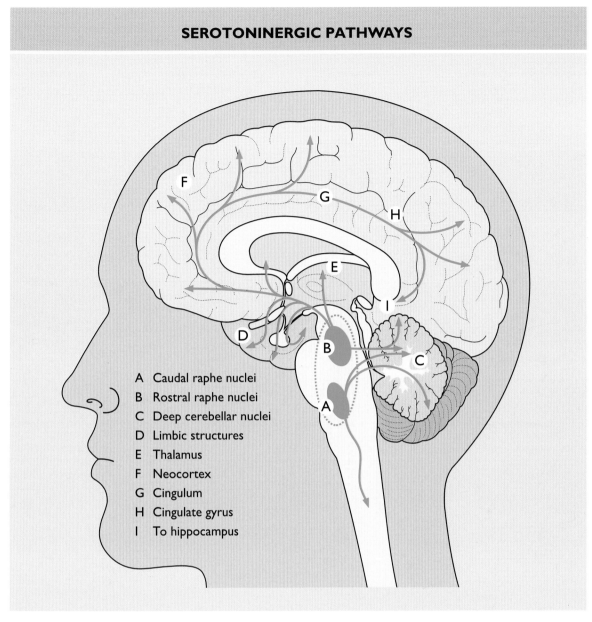

A Caudal raphe nuclei
B Rostral raphe nuclei
C Deep cerebellar nuclei
D Limbic structures
E Thalamus
F Neocortex
G Cingulum
H Cingulate gyrus
I   To hippocampus

Figure 4.10 Representation of the primary serotonin-containing tracts in the human brain. Arising from the raphe nuclei these cells project to all cortical gray matter, with additional tracts to the basal ganglia and the cerebellum

More than nine distinct serotonin (5-HT) receptors have been identified. The 5-HT$_{1A}$, 5-HT$_{2A}$, 5-HT$_{2C}$, and 5-HT$_3$ receptors have been most extensively studied. The major site of serotonergic cell bodies is in the area of the upper pons and midbrain. The classic areas for 5-HT-containing neurons are the median and dorsal raphe nuclei. The neurons from the raphe nuclei project to the basal ganglia and various parts of the limbic system, and have a wide distribution throughout the cerebral cortices in addition to cerebellar connections (Figure 4.10). All the 5-HT receptors identified to date are G-protein coupled receptors, except the 5-HT$_3$ receptor, which is a ligand gated Na$^+$/K$^+$ channel.

5-HT is synthesized from tryptophan by tryptophan hydroxylase, and the supply of tryptophan is the rate-limiting step in the

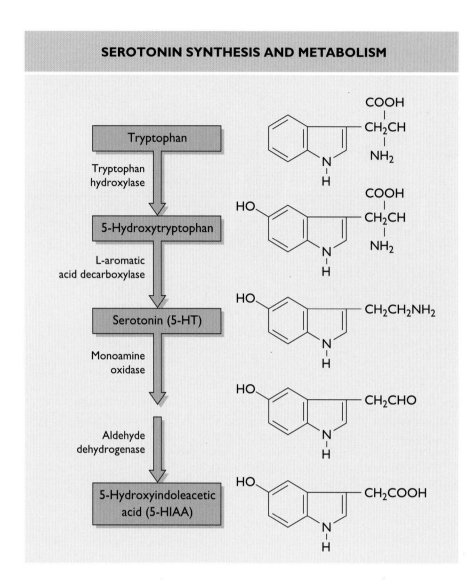

SEROTONIN SYNTHESIS AND METABOLISM

Tryptophan

Tryptophan hydroxylase

5-Hydroxytryptophan

L-aromatic acid decarboxylase

Serotonin (5-HT)

Monoamine oxidase

Aldehyde dehydrogenase

5-Hydroxyindoleacetic acid (5-HIAA)

Figure 4.11 The rate-limiting step for serotonin synthesis is the availability of the precursor tryptophan. Tryptophan hydroxylase is the rate limiting enzyme. Serotonin in the CNS is primarily metabolized by monoamine oxidase. The primary metabolite is 5-hydroxyindoleacetic acid

synthesis of 5-HT (Figure 4.11). 5-HT is primarily broken down by monoamine oxidase and the primary metabolite is 5-HIAA.

Other neurotransmitters

Recent efforts have been directed towards finding an alternative neurochemical target in schizophrenia. The first of these that should be considered is gamma aminobutyric acid (GABA). GABA appears to have a regulatory role on dopaminergic function. The balance of evidence tends to suggest that GABA decreases dopaminergic firing. This links with human postmortem data indicating that GABAergic reductions correlate with increased dopamine concentrations[19,20]. Thus, it is possible that in schizophrenia there is a reduction in GABAergic function which leads to a

dysregulation of dopamine and the production of psychotic symptoms. A more likely candidate, however, appears to be the glutamatergic system. Glutamatergic dysfunction, particularly at the level of the N-methyl-D-aspartate (NMDA) receptor, has also been implicated in the pathophysiology of schizophrenia. Drugs which are antagonistic at the NMDA receptor, such as ketamine and phencyclidine, produce in healthy volunteers, both the positive, negative and neurocognitive symptoms that are characteristic of schizophrenia[21]. There is evidence that the pro-psychotic effects of these drugs may be mediated via an increase in the release of glutamate acting on non-NMDA receptors[22].

If the function of NMDA receptors themselves is decreased this may remove the glutamatergic

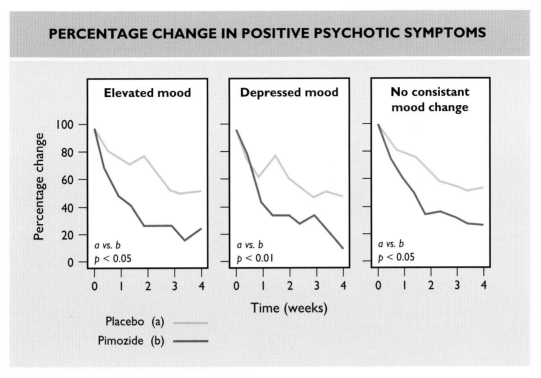

Figure 4.12 Change in positive psychotic symptoms in patients randomized to either the antipsychotic pimozide or to placebo. The groups were subdivided on the basis of the presence of elevated mood, depressed mood or no consistent mood change. The fact that pimozide significantly reduced positive psychotic symptoms in all three groups provided evidence that the 'neuroleptics' are in fact antipsychotic rather than 'anti-schizophrenic'. Figure reproduced with permission from Johnstone EC, Crow TJ, Frith CD, Owens DG. The Northwick Park "functional" psychosis study: diagnosis and treatment response. *Lancet* 1988;2:119–25

drive to inhibitory GABAergic neurons which further regulate the excitatory neurons acting on areas such as the frontal cortex and the limbic regions. Thus, with decreased inhibitory control these neurons may increase firing in these areas and produce psychotic symptoms[23]. Thus, reducing glutamate release at all glutamate receptors may also have a role in improving symptoms in schizophrenia.

EFFICACY OF ANTIPSYCHOTICS IN THE ACUTE PHASE OF TREATMENT

The best known large-scale clinical trial, which gives a good idea of the treatment effect to be expected with antipsychotics, was carried out by the National Institutes of Mental Health, in the USA[24]. This study involved four treatment groups (chlorpromazine, thioridazine, fluphenazine and placebo) with 90 randomly allocated subjects in each. The subjects were treated for 6 weeks and rated on 14 different symptoms in addition to global clinical improvement. In this study 75% of subjects in the chlorpromazine, thioridazine and fluphenazine groups showed significant improvement, 5% failed to be helped and 2% deteriorated. In the placebo group only 25% of patients showed significant improvement, and over 50% were unchanged or worse.

Johnstone and co-workers[25], showed that pimozide was antipsychotic (i.e. reducing the positive symptoms of psychosis) in patients with 'functional' psychosis, regardless of whether the patients had prominent manic or depressive symptoms or were euthymic. This proved that 'neuroleptics', as they were then popularly called, were truly antipsychotic rather than simply antischizophrenic (Figure 4.12).

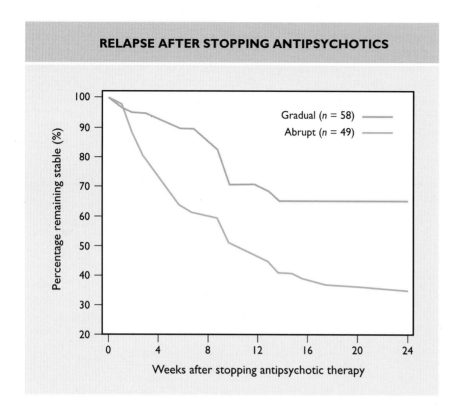

RELAPSE AFTER STOPPING ANTIPSYCHOTICS

Gradual (*n* = 58)
Abrupt (*n* = 49)

Percentage remaining stable (%)

Weeks after stopping antipsychotic therapy

Figure 4.13 The upper line represents the percentage of patients with schizophrenia who remained stable after gradual reduction of antipsychotic medication. The lower line represents patients whose medication was abruptly stopped. These results indicate that abrupt cessation of antipsychotic medication produces a much higher risk of relapse in schizophrenia than a gradual reduction. Figure reproduced with permission from Viguera AC, Baldessarini RJ, Hegarty JD, *et al*. Clinical risk following abrupt and gradual withdrawal of maintenance neuroleptic treatment. *Arch Gen Psychiatry* 1997;54: 49–55

Davis and Andriukaitis[26] performed a meta-analysis using the trials involving chlorpromazine, to investigate the relationship between dose and clinical effect. They noted that a threshold of 400 mg chlorpromazine was required. This was based on the fact that in 31 trials using a dose of ≥400 mg chlorpromazine/day, only one trial failed to show that chlorpromazine was more effective than the non-antipsychotic reference treatment, whereas in the 31 trials using a dose < 400 mg of chlorpromazine, 19 had failed to show a significant effect.

No comparative trials have shown a consistent superiority in any treatment outcome for one conventional or typical antipsychotic over another in the acute treatment of schizophrenia[27].

PHARMACOTHERAPY AS MAINTENANCE TREATMENT IN SCHIZOPHRENIA

Although it is widely accepted that antipsychotic medication is the mainstay of treatment in acute schizophrenia, its role in long-term maintenance has been more contentious. Nevertheless, the importance of maintenance drug therapy in the treatment of chronic schizophrenia has been evident since the early 1960s.

Initial studies indicated that between one-half and two-thirds of patients with schizophrenia who were stable on medication relapsed following cessation of maintenance pharmacological therapy, compared with between 5 and 30% of the patients maintained on medication[28–30].

In a review of 66 studies from 1958 to 1993, Gilbert and colleagues[31] noted that relapse rate in the medication withdrawal groups was 53.2% (follow-up 6.3–9.7 months) compared with 15.6% (follow-up 7.9 months) in the maintenance groups. There was also a positive relationship between risk of relapse and length of follow-up. Viguera and colleagues[32] investigated the relationship between gradual (last depot injection or tailing off over 3 weeks or more) and abrupt medication discontinuation. They noted a cumulative relapse rate of about 46% at 6 months and 56.2% at 24 months of follow-up in patients whose medication was stopped abruptly. They calculated that in patients whose medication was

Table 4.2 Results of four studies comparing continuous medication treatment with 'targeted' or 'crisis' medication treatment. In the latter condition the patients only received medication when psychotic symptoms appeared and medication was stopped when these symptoms had resolved. Treatment was 24 months in all studies. As can be seen, although the targeted/crisis groups received lower total doses of medication they were significantly more likely to have a relapse of their psychotic illness than patients receiving continuous medication. Table adapted with permission from reference 33

Study characteristics	Herz et al. (1991)[35]	Carpenter et al. (1990)[36]	Jolley et al. (1990)[37]	Gaebel et al. (1993)[38]
Number	101	116	54	365
Patient population	outpatients	recently discharged	outpatients	recently hospitalized
Stabilization	3 months	8 weeks	6 months	3 months post-discharge
Psychosocial support	weekly support groups	individual case managers	monthly RN/MD visits	special outpatient clinics
Control features	random/double-blind	random/non-blind	random/fluphenazine decanoate double-blind	random/non-blind
Dosage				
Continued	290*	1.7**	1616†	208††
Targeted early	150	1.0	298	91
Targeted crisis	–	–	–	118
12-month relapse (%)				
Continued	10	33	9	15
Targeted early	29	55	22	35
24-month relapse (%)				
Continued	17	39	14	23
Targeted early	36	62	54	49

*mg/day expressed in chlorpromazine (CPZ) eqivalents; **1 = low, e.g. <300 mg CPZ; 2 = moderate, e.g. 301–600 mg/day; †mean total dose expressed in haloperidol equivalents; ††cumulative dosage over 2 years in 1000 g CPZ equivalents

stopped gradually, the relapse rate at 6 months was halved. Fifty percent of in-patients had relapsed by 5 months after cessation of medication, whilst in their out-patient group relapse rates remained less than 50% to 4 years' follow-up (Figure 4.13).

Thus, findings from medication discontinuation studies have conclusively shown that, as a group patients with schizophrenia fare better if they receive antipsychotic medication. However, prolonged use of antipsychotic medication, particularly the older typical antipsychotics, carries a high risk of adverse effects, particularly tardive dyskinesia. In order to minimize the risk of these events, much recent work has focused on the use of low-dose medication regimes.

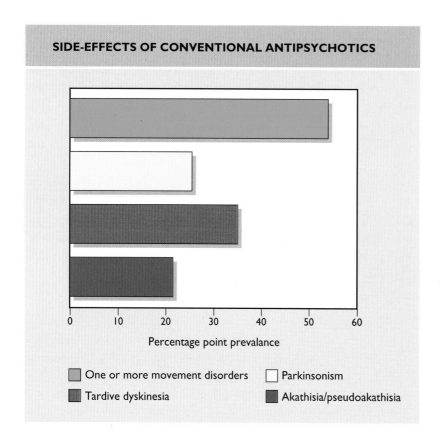

SIDE-EFFECTS OF CONVENTIONAL ANTIPSYCHOTICS

Percentage point prevalance

- One or more movement disorders
- Parkinsonism
- Tardive dyskinesia
- Akathisia/pseudoakathisia

Figure 4.14 Graphical representation of the point prevalence of extrapyramidal side-effects in 88% of all known schizophrenics living in Nithsdale, Southwest Scotland (n = 146), treated with conventional antipsychotics. There was no relationship between antipsychotic plasma levels and akathisia, parkinsonism or tardive dyskinesia. Figure reproduced with permission from McCreadie RG. Robertson LJ. Wiles DH. The Nithsdale schizophrenia surveys. IX: Akathisia, parkinsonism, tardive dyskinesia and plasma neuroleptic levels. *Br J Psychiatry* 1992;160:793–9

Low-dose antipsychotics

The rationale underlying the use of low-dose strategies is that significantly lower doses of medication are required for the maintenance, as opposed to the acute treatment, of schizophrenia. This assumes that all major treatment goals have been met for the patients by the time of dose reduction. The two major aims are to ensure that the stability of symptomatic improvement is at least maintained and to minimize the risk of neurological side-effects and secondary negative symptoms caused by higher doses of antipsychotics, particularly typical antipsychotics.

A number of trials have investigated the use of standard doses of depot antipsychotics (between 250–500 mg chlorpromazine equivalents) in comparison with continuous 'low dose' regimes, usually at least 50% less (reviewed in references 33 and 34). On the whole, these studies have indicated that the patients treated with the lower doses of antipsychotics have a higher rate of exacerbations of their psychotic symptoms and

higher rates of relapse. Barbui and colleagues[34] quoted a relative risk of relapse of 45–65% in the low-dose groups at 12 months' follow-up; with the relapse rate highest in the group with the lowest dose (50 mg chlorpromazine equivalents/day).

Intermittent or targeted medication

This treatment strategy is based on the assumption that patients can be maintained with intermittently administered low doses of antipsychotics. To summarize the results from the main published studies[35–38], it appears that patients receiving intermittent targeted therapy while receiving less medication than those on continuous therapy, have a higher rate of relapse and may have a higher rate of re-hospitalization. At 2 years there is little difference in social functioning or psychopathology between the two groups. However, because of the increased risk of relapse and hospitalization, intermittent targeted treatment is no longer generally recommended (Table 4.2).

SIDE-EFFECTS OF TYPICAL ANTIPSYCHOTICS

Acute neurological side-effects

Acute neurological side-effects secondary to dopamine D_2 receptor blockade with typical antipsychotics include acute dystonia. This is characterized by fixed muscle postures with spasm, e.g. clenched jaw muscles, protruding tongue, opisthotonos, torticollis, oculogyric crisis (mouth open, head back, eyes staring upwards). It appears within hours to days and young males are most at risk. It should be treated immediately with anticholinergic drugs (procyclidine 5–10 mg or benztropine 50–100 mg) intramuscularly or intravenously. The response is dramatic.

Medium-term neurological side-effects

Medium-term neurological side-effects due to D_2 blockade include akathisia and parkinsonism (Figure 4.14)[39]. Akathisia is an inner and motor, generally lower limb, restlessness. It is usually experienced as very distressing by the patient, and can lead to increased disturbance. Treatment is by reducing the neuroleptic dose and/or propranolol, not with anticholinergics. Akathisia usually appears within hours to days. Parkinsonism is due to blockade of D_2 receptors in the basal ganglia. The classical features are a mask-like facies, tremor, rigidity, festinant gait and bradykinesia. It appears after a few days to weeks and treatment involves use of anticholinergic drugs (procyclidine, orphenadrine), reduction in antipsychotic dose, or switching to an 'atypical' antipsychotic which is less likely to produce such extrapyramidal symptoms (Figure 4.15).

Chronic neurological side-effects

The chronic neurological side-effects due to D_2 blockade are tardive dyskinesia and tardive dystonia. Tardive dyskinesia is usually manifested as orofacial dyskinesia and the patient exhibits lip smacking and tongue rotating. Tardive dystonia appears as choreoathetoid movements of the head, neck and trunk. It appears after months to years. There is an increased risk of tardive dyskinesia in older patients, females, the edentulous and patients with organic brain damage. With chronic use of antipsychotics, 20% or more of patients will develop tardive dyskinesia. Although there is no clear relationship with duration or total dose of treatment, or class of antipsychotic used there is a cumulatively increased risk with length of exposure (Figure 4.16)[40]. Increasing the dose may temporarily alleviate symptoms, and reducing the dose may exacerbate them. Clozapine, olanzapine and quetiapine have been shown to improve symptoms, and with risperidone and amisulpride, have a lower propensity to cause tardive dyskinesia.

Neuroendocrine effects

The effect of D_2 blockade on the neuroendocrine system produces hyperprolactinemia by reducing the negative feedback on the anterior pituitary. High serum levels of prolactin produce galactorrhea, amenorrhea and infertility.

Idiosyncratic effects

The most life-threatening side-effect of neuroleptic use is neuroleptic malignant syndrome (NMS). This is thought to be due to derangement of dopaminergic function, but the precise pathophysiology is unknown. Symptoms include hyperthermia, muscle rigidity, autonomic instability and fluctuating consciousness. It is an idiosyncratic reaction. The diagnosis is often missed in the early stages, but a raised level of creatine phosphokinase is often seen. It can occur at any time. The untreated mortality rate is 20% and therefore immediate medical treatment is required. Bromocriptine (a D_1/D_2 agonist) and dantrolene (a skeletal muscle relaxant) are used to reverse dopamine blockade and for muscular rigidity, respectively. The management includes supportive treatment for dehydration and high temperature. Renal failure from rhabdomyolysis is the major complication and cause of mortality. NMS can recur on reintroduction of antipsychotics; it is therefore recommended to wait at least 2 months and introduce a drug of a different class at the lowest effective dose.

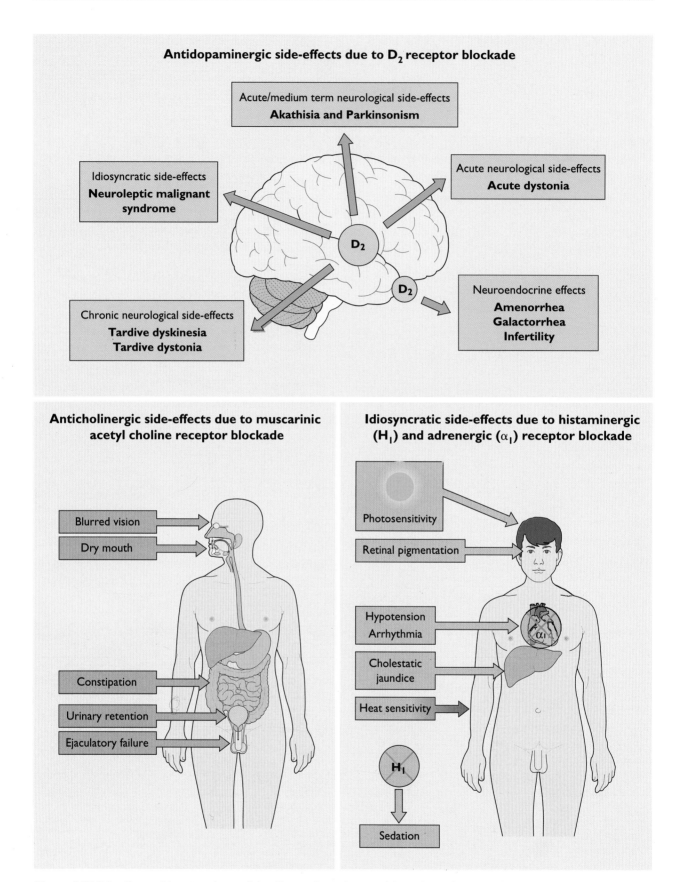

Antidopaminergic side-effects due to D₂ receptor blockade

Acute/medium term neurological side-effects
Akathisia and Parkinsonism

Idiosyncratic side-effects
Neuroleptic malignant syndrome

Acute neurological side-effects
Acute dystonia

D₂

D₂

Chronic neurological side-effects
**Tardive dyskinesia
Tardive dystonia**

Neuroendocrine effects
**Amenorrhea
Galactorrhea
Infertility**

Anticholinergic side-effects due to muscarinic acetyl choline receptor blockade

Blurred vision

Dry mouth

Constipation

Urinary retention

Ejaculatory failure

Idiosyncratic side-effects due to histaminergic (H₁) and adrenergic (α₁) receptor blockade

Photosensitivity

Retinal pigmentation

Hypotension
Arrhythmia

Cholestatic jaundice

Heat sensitivity

α₁

H₁

Sedation

Figure 4.15 Side-effects with antipsychotics. Side-effects will vary between drugs depending on their receptor profile. In general as all antipsychotics produce some degree of dopamine D₂ receptor blockade they are all likely to produce neurological side-effects above a certain dose, with the exception of clozapine and quetiapine

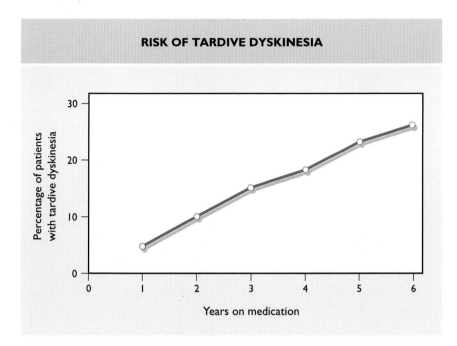

RISK OF TARDIVE DYSKINESIA

Years on medication

Figure 4.16 With prolonged exposure to conventional antipsychotics there is a cumulative risk of tardive dyskinesia with time. Figure reproduced with permission from Glazer WM, Morgenstern H, Doucette JT. Predicting the long-term risk of tardive dyskinesia in out-patients maintained on neuroleptic medications. *J Clin Psychiatry* 1993;54:133–9

Anticholinergic side-effects include a dry mouth (hypersalivation with clozapine), difficulty urinating or retention, constipation, blurred vision and ejaculatory failure. Profound muscarinic blockade may produce a toxic confusional state.

The **sedative effects** of antipsychotics are primarily produced by the blockade of histamine-1 receptors. Side-effects due to α-**adrenergic blockade** include postural hypotension, cardiac arrhythmias and impotence.

Some side-effects may be due to **autoimmune reactions** such as urticaria, dermatitis and rashes. Dermal photosensitivity and a gray/blue/purple skin tinge are more commonly seen with the phenothiazines, as are the conjunctival, corneolenticular and retinal pigmentation sometimes reported. Cholestatic jaundice due to a hypersensitivity reaction is now rarely seen with chlorpromazine and was possibly due to an impurity.

Weight gain is also frequently seen with a wide variety of antipsychotics. This may be due to increased appetite, and although the mechanism is unclear, it may be due to a combination of histamine-1 and 5-HT_{2C} receptor blockade.

Cardiac conduction effects of antipsychotics

Recently, concern has grown over the ability of antipsychotic medications to produce changes in cardiac conduction. QT_C interval prolongation is the most widely reported conduction deficit. This first came to attention after sudden deaths secondary to arrhythmias with pimozide. The UK Committee for the Safety of Medicines' (CSM) advice about pimozide is that all patients should have an electrocardiogram (ECG) prior to starting treatment and patients with a known arrhythmia or prolonged QT interval should not receive the drug. Sertindole, an atypical antipsychotic, was voluntarily suspended from sale by its manufacturers in 1997 after similar concerns. Most recently the CSM has advised on restrictions to the use of thioridazine and droperidol as these medications produce the most profound QT_C prolongations[41].

The QT interval on the standard ECG represents the interval between the end of ventricular depolarization and the end of cardiac repolarization. The 'c' in QT_C indicates that the QT value quoted has been corrected for cardiac rate. It is thought that prolongation of this interval increases the risk of a potentially fatal ventricular arrhythmia known as torsade-de-pointes.

The mechanism of this is becoming clearer and implicates the blockade of the delayed rectifier potassium channel (I(kr)). Blockade of this receptor in the heart prolongs cardiac repolarizaton and thus the QT_C interval. It is known that drugs most

Table 4.3 Amisulpride *vs.* reference antipsychotics – selectivity for recombinant human D_2/D_3 receptor subtypes. Amisulpride only has appreciable affinity for D_2 and D_3 receptors in contrast to the other antipsychotics in this table. It has relatively high affinity for both receptors. The implications of this for amisulpride's mechanism of action and atypicality are hypothesized to involve an increased tendency to bind to presynaptic D_2 and D_2-like receptors. Table reproduced with permission from Schoemaker H, Claustre Y. Fage D, *et al.* Neurochemical characteristics of amisulpride, an atypical dopamine D_2/D_3 receptor antagonist with both presynaptic and limbic selectivity. *J Pharmacol Exp Ther* 1997;280:83–97

Compound	Positively coupled with adenyl cyclase		Negatively coupled with adenyl cyclase		
	D_1	D_5	D_2	D_3	D_4
Amisulpride	>10000	>10000	2.8	3.2	>1000
Haloperidol	27	48	0.6	3.8	3.8
Clozapine	141	250	80	230	89
Olanzapine	250	–	17	44	–
Risperidone	620	–	3.3	13	–

specifically associated with QT_C interval prolongation bind specifically to the I(kr)[42].

Although there is little consensus as to what represents a 'normal' QT_C it is generally accepted that a QT_C of over 500 ms increases the likelihood of an arrhythmia. When interpreting data on medication-related QT_C prlongation it is important to note that the mean daily QT_C intrasubject variability is 76ms[43].

Other risks factors which increase the likelihood of QT_C prolongation include age over 65 years and co-administration of other drugs associated with cardiac arrythmias, such as tricyclic antidepressants. Safety studies are ongoing with both the newer and the older medications, preliminary data suggests that the newer medications do not differ significantly in their likelihood to prolong the QT_C interval.

THE NEWER 'ATYPICAL' ANTIPSYCHOTICS

The reintroduction of clozapine in the early 1990s and the subsequent release of several new, 'atypical' antipsychotics has increased optimism in the treatment of schizophrenia. As these are likely to be the mainstay of treatment for schizophrenia in the future, it is worthwhile considering them individually (Figure 4.17 and Table 4.3)[44,45].

Clozapine

Clozapine, the prototypical third-generation antipsychotic, has been used since the 1960s for treatment of schizophrenia. However, after reports of several deaths from neutropenia, in most countries clozapine can be used only in patients unresponsive to two other antipsychotics given at an adequate dose for an adequate duration, or those with tardive dyskinesia or severe extrapyramidal symptoms, and only with blood monitoring. Each patient has to be registered and the drug is dispensed only after a normal white cell count. In the UK, a blood count is performed every week for 18 weeks, then every 2 weeks for the next year, and thereafter monthly. In the USA, blood monitoring is weekly throughout treatment. Clozapine is contraindicated for those with previous neutropenia.

Important aspects of clozapine's pharmacology include its low affinity for the D_2 receptor, in comparison with older antipsychotics. Clozapine has higher affinity at the D_1 and D_4 receptors than at the D_2 receptor and also binds to the extrastriatal D_2-like receptor, the D_3 receptor. It is thought that the low incidence of extrapyramidal side-effects is due to the low activity at the D_2 receptor. Clozapine also has antagonistic activity at the $5HT_{1A}$, $5HT_{2A}$, $5HT_{2C}$ and $5HT_3$

COMPARISON OF ABSOLUTE RECEPTOR BINDING AFFINITIES

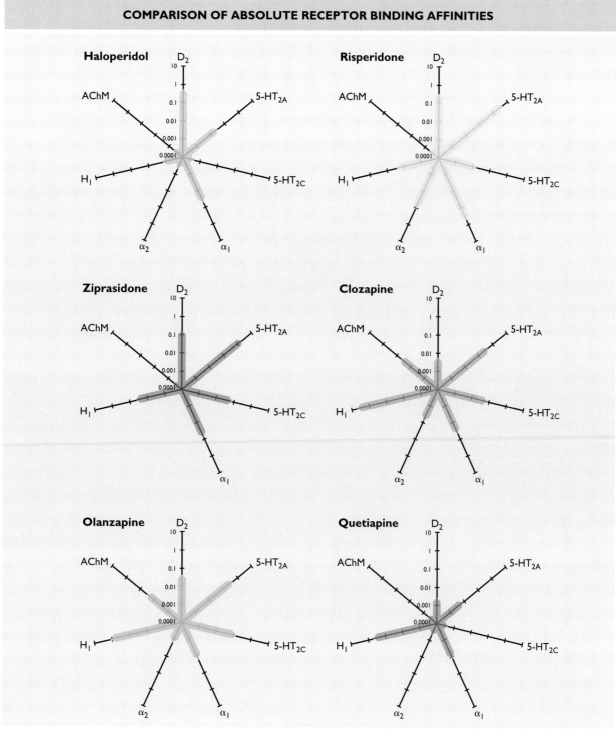

Figure 4.17 A representation of the absolute receptor affinity of haloperidol in comparison with some of the newer 'atypical' antipsychotics drawn from data in reference 112. Each line represents a single receptor, the further along the bar on a given line the higher the affinity of that medication for that receptor. Each of the gradations on the lines represents 10 times greater affinity for that receptor. What can be seen from this is that clozapine, quetiapine and to a lesser extent olanzapine have much lower affinities for the dopamine D_2 receptor than haloperidol. This may be why they are 'atypical' in terms of producing fewer extrapyrimidal side-effects than antipsychotics such as haloperidol. Risperidone and ziprasidone have similar D_2 receptor affinities to haloperidol and yet they too are 'atypical'. It has been hypothesized that very high affinity for the serotonin-2A receptor, (5-HT_{2A}), may underlie the atypicality of ziprasidone and risperidone. Indeed this may be important for 'atypicality' *per se*, as all of the newer medications have a higher affinity for the 5-HT_{2A} than for the D_2 receptor. Amisulpride, by contrast to the medications in this figure, only has appreciable affinity for D_2 and D_3 receptors and has high equipotent affinity for both receptors, as can be seen in Table 4.3. Data from reference 45

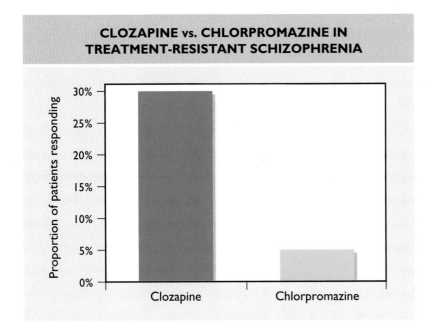

CLOZAPINE vs. CHLORPROMAZINE IN TREATMENT-RESISTANT SCHIZOPHRENIA

Figure 4.18 Comparison of efficacy of clozapine versus chlorpromazine in treatment-resistant schizophrenia. Figure reproduced with permission from Kane J, Honigfeld G, Singer J, Meltzer H. Clozapine for the treatment-resistant schizophrenic: a double blind comparison with chlorpromazine. *Arch Gen Psychiatry* 1988; 45:789–96

receptors. It is postulated that it is the balance between the blockade of these receptors that underlies clozapine's clinical efficacy in improving positive and negative symptomatology. Clozapine is an antagonist at the α_1 receptor but less so at the α_2 receptor, resulting in sedation and hypotension. Clozapine's antagonism at the histamine H_1 receptor adds to the sedative effects and may be, in part, responsible for weight gain. Other side-effects include hypersalivation, tachycardia, sedation and hypotension. More rarely, clozapine can produce seizures (approximately 1%) and blood dyscrasias (< 1–2%). The risk of neutropenia is 1–2%, and in most cases is reversible. The majority of cases (83%) occur within the first 20 weeks of treatment. Risk of agranulocytosis decreases to 0.07% after the first year of treatment. Agranulocytosis probably results from toxic and immunological factors (reviewed in reference 46). It is this last potentially fatal side-effect that has led to the limits on the use of clozapine and the requirement for blood monitoring in patients receiving clozapine. Interestingly, clozapine does not increase serum prolactin.

Clozapine is the most effective treatment for schizophrenic patients refractory to other therapies, and improves both positive and negative symptoms. In non-comparative studies, clozapine has led to > 15% improvement in baseline ratings in 30–70% of previously treatment-refractory patients after 2–6 months of treatment (reviewed in reference 46). In comparison to chlorpromazine[47–49] (Figure 4.18), haloperidol[50] or fluphenazine[51], clozapine shows a 30–100% response rate, versus a 4–17% rate for the comparator, when administered to patients resistant to previous treatment with classical antipsychotics.

Clozapine has been investigated in few randomized controlled trials of maintenance therapy. This is due to the restrictions imposed on its use. In one of the few studies published, Essock and co-workers[52] followed up a sample of 227 patients randomized to either clozapine or treatment as usual. They reported that those treated with clozapine had significantly greater reductions in side-effects, disruptiveness, hospitalization and readmission after discharge. Furthermore, the clinical efficacy of clozapine in relapse prevention is well established, naturalistically, at 1–2 years of treatment and there have been reports of good maintenance efficacy for up to 17 years of treatment (for review see reference 46).

Risperidone

This drug has high affinity for the 5-HT_{2A} receptor, with a similar affinity at the D_2 receptor to most typical antipsychotics. In the acute phase of treatment, risperidone appears as effective as haloperidol in terms of improvement in positive and secondary negative symptom scores[53].

The optimal dose of risperidone appears to be between 4 and 6 mg/day. At doses higher than 8–12 mg/day risperidone can cause extrapyramidal side-effects of tremor, rigidity and restlessness, with a similar frequency to typical antipsychotics. Risperidone can increase serum prolactin which may lead to sexual dysfunction.

Risperidone has been assessed for long-term efficacy and safety in a number of long-term open-label studies. Earlier data suggested that long-term therapy with risperidone was associated with a meaningful reduction in psychopathology, amelioration of extrapyrimidal side-effects (EPS) and improved social functioning from baseline measures or against placebo.

More recently a meta-analysis of eleven of the risperidone/conventional antipsychotic comparator randomized controlled trials was performed[54]. The author reported that slightly but significantly more patients on risperidone showed clinical improvement than with comparison antipsychotics (57% vs. 52%) and used significantly less medication for EPS (29.1% vs. 33.9%).

Olanzapine

A more broad-spectrum atypical antipsychotic, olanzapine has a side-effect profile similar to that of clozapine but with a higher incidence of extrapyrimidal side-effects at doses above 20 mg/day. Olanzapine also demonstrates antagonistic effects at a wide range of receptors, but has a higher affinity for D_2 and 5-HT_{2A} receptors than clozapine and a lower affinity at the D_1 receptor subtype. In acute-phase studies, olanzapine is efficacious for positive and secondary negative symptoms and was superior to haloperidol on overall improvement according to the Brief Psychiatric Rating Scale (BPRS)[55] and every other secondary measure.

Standard-dose olanzapine (5–15 mg/day) has been shown to be an effective maintenance treatment for schizophrenia in comparison with placebo[56]. The estimated 1-year risk of relapse with olanzapine was 19.6–28.6% for standard-dose olanzapine in comparison with a 69.9% risk of relapse with placebo. Initial data from a meta-analysis of three studies using haloperidol-treated patients as a test group, indicated that 80.3% of patients receiving olanzapine maintained their response at 1 year in comparison with 72% for haloperidol-treated patients[57].

Quetiapine

Another broader-spectrum atypical, quetiapine has a similar receptor binding profile to clozapine, but with relatively lower affinity for all receptors and virtually no affinity for muscarinic receptors. Quetiapine is effective in acute phase studies for the treatment of positive and secondary negative symptoms. Initial randomized controlled trials indicated that quetiapine (250–750 mg, $n=96$) was more effective than placebo ($n=96$) and that this efficacy was not seen at doses of less than 250 mg/day of quetiapine[58]. In comparison with chlorpromazine, response rates to quetiapine were similar across all symptom domains[59]. Response rates between haloperidol- and quetiapine-treated groups are also similar[60].

In all of these studies, the rates of EPS with quetiapine were similar to those seen in placebo-treated groups and significantly lower than in conventional antipsychotic comparator groups. Most common side-effects are somnolence and dry mouth. Quetiapine demonstrates a lower potential to cause weight gain than clozapine and olanzapine, and does not increase serum prolactin[61].

In long-term studies, quetiapine was well tolerated with up to 75% of respondents to a questionnaire denying any side-effects from quetiapine[62].

Amisulpride

In contrast to all the other newer antipsychotics, amisulpride only has effects on the dopamine D_2 and D_3 receptors, where it is a potent antagonist. In animal models at lower doses, amisulpride appears to bind preferentially to presynaptic D_2 receptors[64], and at projected therapeutic levels it also appears to be selective, in a neurochemical imaging study in humans, for limbic D_2 and D_3 receptors[63]. It has a similar efficacy to haloperidol for positive symptoms in acute exacerbations of schizophrenia[64–67], with a projected optimum dose in this group of between 400 and 800 mg/day[66]. Some studies at this dose range have reported a significantly greater efficacy for amisulpride in comparison with placebo for treating the negative symptoms of schizophrenia[65,66].

In all of the studies above, amisulpride has a significantly lower incidence of extrapyramidal side-effects, at doses below 1200 mg/day, than haloperidol. Amisulpride may cause less weight gain than other atypical antipsychotics but it does increase plasma prolactin[68,69].

In a 12-month trial of amisulpride 200–800 mg/day versus haloperidol 5–20 mg/day, amisulpride showed enhanced efficacy for positive and negative symptoms in comparison with haloperidol. Those treated with amisulpride had significantly greater improvement in quality of life and significantly fewer extrapyramidal side-effects. Long-term efficacy and relapse prevention were similar in the amisulpride- and haloperidol-treated groups[70].

Ziprasidone

Ziprasidone has a high $5HT_{2A}/D_2$ receptor blockade ratio and a similarly high affinity for the $5HT_{2A}$ receptor to risperidone and sertindole. It is an agonist at the $5HT_{1A}$ receptor. Ziprasidone also has potent affinity for D_3 and moderate affinity for D_4 receptors. It exhibits weak serotonin and noradrenergic reuptake inhibition.

Ziprasidone appears to have relatively low levels of side-effects. These may include somnolence and headache, but results of full clinical studies remain to be published.

An initial clinical trial of ziprasidone versus haloperidol 15 mg/day over 4 weeks suggested that ziprasidone 160 mg/day was as effective as haloperidol at reducing positive symptom scores, but produced fewer side-effects[71]. In two placebo-controlled trials lasting 4 and 6 weeks, respectively[72,73], the pooled data indicated that ziprasidone 80–160 mg was consistently significantly more effective than placebo and lower doses of ziprasidone. Improvements in positive and negative symptoms were similar in magnitude to those seen in patients treated with risperidone, olanzapine or quetiapine. Interestingly, 160 mg of ziprasidone was associated with a greater than 30% decrease in depressive symptoms in the subgroup of patients with significant depression at the outset of the trials.

Ziprasidone has also been used in a 1-year placebo-controlled trial in order to assess its utility for relapse prevention. A total of 294 patients were studied and randomized to placebo treatment or ziprasidone 40–160 mg/day. At 6 months into the study, 117 patients remained on ziprasidone and 23 on placebo. Of these, only 6% of the ziprasidone-treated patients had experienced an exacerbation of their symptoms over the subsequent 6 months, in comparison with 35% in the placebo-treated group[74].

NEW ANTIPSYCHOTICS CURRENTLY IN PHASE III CLINICAL TRIALS

Iloperidone

Iloperidone is a benzisoxazole derivative and is therefore from the same chemical class as risperidone. As for risperidone, iloperidone has a high affinity for the $5\text{-}HT_{2A}$ receptor and a lower affinity for the D_2 receptor, although in absolute terms its affinity for the D_2 receptor is of a similar order of magnitude to haloperidol and risperidone. Relative to other newer antipsychotics iloperidone has a higher affinity for $5\text{-}HT_{1A}$ receptors and lower affinity for $5\text{-}HT_{2C}$ receptors[75]. It also has high affinity for α_1 receptors but no affinity for acetylcholine muscarinic M_1 receptors.

In early phase II placebo controlled trials, iloperidone at 8 mg per day was superior to placebo in improving positive and negative symptoms with EPS at placebo levels. The most frequently described side-effects were dizziness, postural hypotension and nausea[76].

A large scale multicenter trial comparing iloperidone 4 mg, 8 mg and 12 mg with haloperidol 15 mg per day and placebo in a total of 621 patients over 42 days has recently been completed[77]. Initial data indicates clinical response similar to haloperidol but with significantly lower rates of EPS (similar to placebo).

Aripiprazole

Aripiprazole is a quinolinone derivative and differs from other novel antipsychotics in that rather than being an antagonist at dopamine receptors, it appears to be a high affinity partial agonist at presynaptic D_2 receptors but exhibits antagonist effects on postsynaptic D_2 receptors[78]. It has low affinity for D_3 and D_4 receptors and no appreciable affinity for D_1-like receptors. Its affinity for $5-HT_{2A}$ receptors is low and of a similar magnitude to that of clozapine.

In phase II clinical studies, aripiprazole is significantly superior to placebo at improving the total score of the PANSS[79]. A recently completed phase III clinical trial compared aripiprazole 15 mg or 30 mg per day with haloperidol 10 mg per day and placebo in a total of 414 patients for 28 days. The preliminary results from this study show that both doses of aripiprazole are significantly better than placebo at improving PANSS total score and equivalent to haloperidol. Aripiprazole at both doses lead to placebo rates of EPS which is significantly lower than the rate seen in the patients treated with haloperidol[80].

ADVERSE EVENTS OF ATYPICAL ANTIPSYCHOTICS

The issue of side-effects or adverse events is closely linked to tolerability and acceptability and therefore to both compliance and relapse prevention. Often the most debilitating and obvious side-effects of conventional antipsychotics are motor.

As described above, all of the newer antipsychotics demonstrate a lower propensity to cause EPS at clinically effective doses. There is increasing evidence that these drugs may additionally provide benefits for patients who suffer from akathisia and tardive dyskinesia.

Indeed, it is in the area of tardive dyskinesias that clozapine appears to have its most marked effect. Lieberman and associates[81] reported a 50% reduction of symptoms over 28 months of treatment in 43% of patients, and Gerlach and Peacock[82] reported a resolution of tardive dyskinesia in 54% of patients after 5 years of clozapine treatment. Furthermore, Tamminga and colleagues[83] reported a significant difference in reduction of tardive dyskinesia scores in a clozapine group versus a haloperidol-treated group and that this difference began after about 4 months of treatment. There have also been case reports that switching to clozapine has been effective in reducing tardive dystonia[84].

Initial data from the studies quoted above on the newer antipsychotics indicates that they too produce very low rates of tardive dyskinesia. The rate of other side-effects may vary between each of the newer drugs, although fully adequate comparison studies remain to be published (Table 4.4)[85].

Negative symptoms

It is claimed that clozapine has an almost unique action against the negative symptoms of schizophrenia, out of proportion to its effect on positive symptoms[86], but the evidence for this is by no means clear. Tandon and associates[87] found that the improvement in negative symptoms covaried with the improvement in positive symptoms, and Hagger and co-workers[88] found no improvement in negative symptoms. A more recent finding is that in comparison with haloperidol, clozapine had a significant effect on negative symptoms in patients with non-deficit schizophrenia, but not in those with deficit schizophrenia, i.e. those with enduring negative symptoms[89,90]. It has therefore been suggested that clozapine's apparently beneficial effect on negative symptoms may simply be a reflection of its reduced tendency to cause EPS[91]. The weight of current evidence suggests that

Table 4.4 Qualitative comparison of the relative side-effects of the newer medications. These will be subject to change over time, as new tolerability data are published and report forms returned. Adapted from reference 85

	Typicals	Clozapine	Risperidone	Olanzapine	Quetiapine	Amisulpride	Ziprasidone
Anticholinergic	±	+++	±	+	±	±	±
Orthostatic hypotension	± to +++	+++	+	±	+	±	±
Prolactin elevation	++ to +++	0	++	±	±	++	±
QT prolongation	± to +	+	± to +	± to +	± to +	±	± to +
Sedation	+ to +++	+++	+	++	++	±	+
Seizures	±	++ to +++	±	±	±	±	±
Weight gain	± to ++	+++	+ to ++	+++	+ to ++	± to +	±

clozapine has an excellent effect on the secondary, but not primary, negative symptoms[92]. All of the newer antipsychotics appear to have an effect on secondary negative symptoms. Most of the available trials have indicated a modest but significant advantage for all of the newer medications over conventional antipsychotics in negative symptom improvement[54,58,87,93].

Amisulpride at low doses (50–300 mg/day) is claimed to have a unique effect in patients with only negative symptoms. In comparison with placebo, these low doses of amisulpride produced significant reductions in negative symptom scores with little change in positive symptom scores[94–96]. However, in a study utilizing a different design but similar patient population, low-dose amisulpride was similar to low-dose haloperidol treatment in terms of negative symptom improvement[97].

Cognition

Neurocognitive deficits that are a core feature of schizophrenia, are apparent at the onset of illness and may deteriorate during the first few years of illness. The older antipsychotics have limited impact on these, although inconsistent long-term improvements have been noted[98,99]. There has been increasing interest in the possibility that the newer antipsychotics may ameliorate these problems which are linked to poor outcome and future unemployment. Clozapine may lead to improvements in attention, memory and executive function over 6–12 months[100]. Risperidone is claimed to improve frontal function and spatial working memory compared with haloperidol[101,102]. Olanzapine is claimed to improve a variety of measures of function including psychomotor speed, verbal fluency and memory[103]. It has recently been reported that quetiapine improves attentional performance to the level of that seen in a matched control group over 2 months of treatment[104]. In a study comparing haloperidol 1 mg and 2 mg and amisulpride 50 mg and 100 mg with placebo in healthy volunteers, the haloperidol-treated groups showed greater cognitive impairment on tasks measuring problem-solving abilites[105].

It is still not clear how relevant the modest improvements or impairments reported in these studies are to long-term outcome.

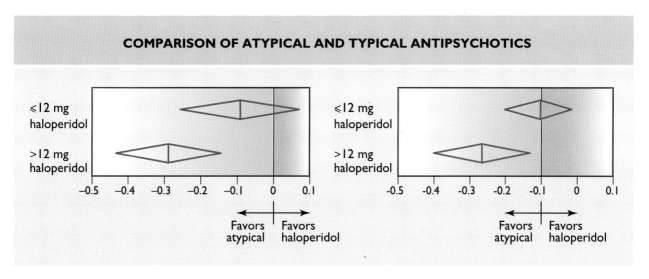

Figure 4.18 Results from a meta-analysis of trials comparing newer atypical antipsychotics and typical antipsychotics (mainly haloperidol). The left graph suggests that the clinical superiority of atypical antipsychotics over typical antipsychotics is lost if lower doses of typical antipsychotics are used (less than 12 mg per day of haloperidol equivalents). The right-hand graph, suggests that any superiority in tolerability for the atypical antipsychotics is similarly lost if patients receive lower doses of typical antipsychotics. These findings and interpretations have been criticized on a number of counts including selection bias in the trials chosen for the meta-analysis, no similar control for the doses of atypicals used and using the drop-out rates from clinical trials as a measure of medication tolerability. Figure reproduced with permission from Geddes J, Freemantle N, Harrison P, Bebbington P. Atypical antipsychotics in the treatment of schizophrenia: systematic overview and meta-regression analysis. *Br Med J* 2000;321:1371–6

Affective symptoms

Patients with schizophrenia are significantly more likely than the general population to suffer from other psychiatric disorders such as depression, and conventional antipsychotics are used to treat other psychotic disorders outside of schizophrenia.

Clozapine has been reported to be effective in patients with treatment-resistant schizoaffective or manic illnesses[106] (see reference 107 for review). In one study, clozapine reduced baseline mania ratings by more than 50% in 72% of a group of patients suffering from either mania or schizoaffective disorder and 32% had a significant improvement in BPRS scores. The latter finding was more frequent in the patients with bipolar disorder and the non-rapid cycling patients[108]. In depressive disorders, clozapine had a more equivocal response. Although it was seemingly effective against depressive symptoms occurring comorbidly with schizophrenia[109], there has been little work showing a particular use for clozapine in treatment-refractory depression[110,111].

Conventional antipsychotics may both improve and contribute towards depressive symptoms. Clozapine reduces both depressive features and suicidality[109]. Risperidone produces significantly greater reduction in anxiety/depression subscales in comparison with haloperidol[52]. Olanzapine has significant antidepressant effects in comparison with haloperidol[112]. Amisulpride (50 mg/day) has been compared with imipramine (100 mg/day) and placebo in patients with dysthymia and major depressive disorder. In this study ($n = 219$), both imipramine and amisulpride produced similar and significant improvements on all rating scales[113]. The implications of this in patients with schizophrenia have yet to be elucidated.

THE FUTURE

Despite the advances in schizophrenia pharmacotherapy since the early 1950s there are still many limitations. EPS make use of high doses of the older typical antipsychotics problematic and often unpleasant for those taking them. Lower doses of 'typicals' and the newer 'atypical' antipsychotics offer benefits in terms of reductions in EPS, but the latter medications are not without their own unpleasant side-effects. In a recent meta-analysis, Geddes and colleagues[114] described that in their analysis of all of the trials of atypical anti-psychotics versus typical antipsychotics there was no treatment advantage for the newer medications over doses of haloperidol below 12 mg/day and no significant difference in total side-effect load (Figure 4.19). Such meta-analyses have, however, come under criticism for obscuring real treatment effects by being overinclusive of available trials[115,116]. Furthermore, a recent critical review of treatment trials with low-dose typical anti-psychotics could find no convincing evidence that there is a low dose of typical antipsychotics which is effective but does not produce EPS[117].

Another failing in the pharmacotherapy of schizophrenia is that there are still 40–50% of patients with schizophrenia who do not have an optimal response to medication, and some 20% who are resistant to all forms of treatment, including clozapine.

Future developments may include a new generation of antipsychotic drugs which are partial agonists (rather than antagonists) at D_2 and D_2-like receptors, such as aripiprazole[78]. As described above, early clinical trials with this medication show good efficacy with placebo rates of EPS[80].

In conjunction with developments in trial methodology, combinations of neurochemical and functional imaging may help to elucidate the neural correlates of treatment response and resistance and allow more rationale therapeutic decisions.

Pharmacogenetics may further help to define the parameters which predict response or non-response to particular medications by analyzing the allelic variations for individual receptors which correlate with response[118].

REFERENCES

1. Carlsson A, Lindqvist M. Effect of chlorpromazine or haloperidol on formation of 3-methoxytyramine and normetanephrine in mouse brain. *Acta Pharmacol Toxicol* 1963;20:140–4

2. Creese I, Burt DR, Snyder SH. Dopamine receptor binding predicts clinical and pharmacological potencies of antischizophrenic drugs. *Science* 1976; 19:481–3

3. Angrist B, van Kammen DP. CNS stimulants as a tool in the study of schizophrenia. *Trends Neurosci* 1984; 7:388–90

4. Lieberman JA, Kane JM, Alvir J. Provocative tests with psychostimulant drugs in schizophrenia. *Psychopharmacology* 1987;91:415–33

5. Laruelle M. Imaging dopamine transmission in schizophrenia. A review and meta-analysis. *Q J Nucl Med* 1998;42:211–21

6. Kapur S, Zipursky R, Jones C, et al. Relationship between dopamine D(2) occupancy, clinical response, and side effects: a double-blind PET study of first-episode schizophrenia. *Am J Psychiatry* 2000;157:514–20

7. Farde L, Nordstrom AL. PET analysis indicates atypical central dopamine receptor occupancy in clozapine-treated patients. *Br J Psychiatry* 1992;17 (Suppl.):30-3

8. Pilowsky LS, Costa DC, Ell PJ, et al. Clozapine, single photon emission tomography, and the D2 dopamine receptor blockade hypothesis of schizophrenia. *Lancet* 1992;340:199–202

9. Broich K, Grunwald F, Kasper S, et al. D₂-dopamine receptor occupancy measured by IBZM-SPECT in relation to extrapyramidal side effects. *Pharmaco-psychiatry* 1998;31:159–62

10. Busatto GF, Kerwin RW. Perspectives on the role of serotonergic mechanisms in the pharmacology of schizophrenia. *J Psychopharmacol* 1997;11:3–12

11. Laruelle M, Abi-Dargham A, Gil R, et al. Increased dopamine transmission in schizophrenia: relation-ship to illness phases. *Biol Psychiatry* 1999;46:56–72

12. Woolley DW, Shaw E. A biological and pharmaco-logical suggestion about certain mental disorders. *Proc Natl Acad Sci USA* 1954;40:228–31

13. Okubo Y, Suhara T, Suzuki K, et al. Serotonin 5-HT₂ receptors in schizophrenic patients studied by positron emission tomography. *Life Sci* 2000;66: 2455–64

14. Verhoeff NP, Meyer JH, Kecojevic A, et al. A voxel-by-voxel analysis of [18F]setoperone PET data shows no substantial serotonin 5-HT(2A) receptor changes in schizophrenia. *Psychiatry Res* 2000;99: 123–35

15. Nordstrom AL, Farde L, Halldin C. High 5-HT$_2$ receptor occupancy in clozapine treated patients demonstrated by PET. *Psychopharmacology* 1993; 110:365–7

16. Travis MJ, Busatto GF, Pilowsky LS, *et al.* 5-HT$_{2A}$ receptor blockade in patients with schizophrenia treated with risperidone or clozapine. A SPET study using the novel 5-HT$_{2A}$ ligand 123I-5-I-R-91150. *Br J Psychiatry* 1998;173:236–41

17. Kapur S, Zipursky RB, Remington G. Clinical and theoretical implications of 5-HT$_2$ and D$_2$ receptor occupancy of clozapine, risperidone, and olanzapine in schizophrenia. *Am J Psychiatry* 1999;156:286–93

18. Travis MJ, Busatto GF, Pilowsky LS, et al. 5-HT2A receptor occupancy in schizophrenic patients: Typical versus atypical antipsychotics. *J Psychopharmacol* 1998;12(Suppl. A54):215

19. Benes FM. The role of stress and dopamine-GABA interactions in the vulnerability for schizophrenia. *J Psychiatr Res* 1997;31:257–75

20. Wassef AA, Dott SG, Harris A, *et al.* Critical review of GABA-ergic drugs in the treatment of schizophrenia. *J Clin Psychopharmacol* 1999;19:222–32

21. Krystal JH, Karper LP, Seibyl JP, *et al.* Subanesthetic effects of the noncompetitive NMDA antagonist, ketamine, in humans. Psychotomimetic, perceptual, cognitive, and neuroendocrine responses. *Arch Gen Psychiatry* 1994;51:199–214

22. Moghaddam B, Adams B, Verma A, Daly D. Activation of glutamatergic neurotransmission by ketamine: a novel step in the pathway from NMDA receptor blockade to dopaminergic and cognitive disruptions associated with the prefrontal cortex. *J Neurosci* 1997;17:2921–7

23. Farber NB, Newcomer JW, Olney JW. The glutamate synapse in neuropsychiatric disorders. Focus on schizophrenia and Alzheimer's disease. *Prog Brain Res* 1998;116:421–37

24. National Institutes of Mental Health. Phenothiazine treatment in schizophrenia. *Arch Gen Psychiatry* 1964;10:246–26

25. Johnstone EC, Crow TJ, Frith CD, Owens DG. The Northwick Park "functional" psychosis study: diagnosis and treatment response. *Lancet* 1988;2:119–25

26. Davis JM, Andriukaitis S. The natural course of schizophrenia and effective maintainence treatment. *J Clin Psychopharmacol* 1986;6(Suppl.):2–10

27. Marder SR, Wirsching WC, van Putten T. Drug treatment of schizophrenia. Overview of recent research. *Schizoph Res* 1991;4:81–90

28. Caffey EM, Diamond LS, Frank TV, *et al.* Discontinuation or reduction of chemotherapy in chronic schizophrenics. *J Chronic Dis* 1964;17: 347–58

29. Hogarty GE, Goldberg SC, Schooler NR, *et al.* Drug and sociotherapy in the aftercare of schizophrenic patients. II: two year relapse rates. *Arch Gen Psychiatry* 1974;31:603–8

30. Davis JM. Overview: maintenance therapy in psychiatry – I. Schizophrenia. *Am J Psychiatry* 1975; 132:1237–45

31. Gilbert PL, Harris J, McAdams LA, Jeste DV. Neuroleptic withdrawal in schizophrenic patients. *Arch Gen Psychiatry* 1995;52:173–88

32. Viguera AC, Baldessarini RJ, Hegarty JD, *et al.* Clinical Risk following abrupt and gradual withdrawal of maintenance neuroleptic treatment. *Arch Gen Psychiatry* 1997;54:49–55

33. Schooler NA. Reducing dosage in maintainence treatment of schizophrenia. *Br J Psychiatry* 1993; 163(Suppl. 22):58–65

34. Barbui C, Saraceno B, Liberati A, Garattini S. Low-dose neuroleptic therapy and relapse in schizophrenia: metaanalysis of randomised controlled trials. *Eur Psychiatry* 1996;11:306–13

35. Herz MI, Glazer WM, Mostert MA, *et al.* Intermittent vs maintenance medication in schizophrenia. Two-year results. *Arch Gen Psychiatry* 1991;48:333–9

36. Carpenter WT Jr, Hanlon TE, Heinrichs DW, Summerfelt AT. Continuous versus targeted medication in schizophrenic outpatients: outcome results [erratum appears in *Am J Psychiatry* 1991; 148:819]. *Am J Psychiatry* 1990;147:1138–48

37. Jolley AG, Hirsch SR, Morrison E, *et al.* Trial of brief intermittent neuroleptic prophylaxis for selected schizophrenic outpatients: clinical and social outcome at two years. *Br Med J* 1990;301:837–42

38. Gaebel W, Frick U, Kopcke W, *et al.* Early neuroleptic intervention in schizophrenia: are prodromal symptoms valid predictors of relapse? *Br J Psychiatry* 1993;21(Suppl.):8–12

39. McCreadie RG, Robertson LJ, Wiles DH. The Nithsdale schizophrenia surveys. IX: Akathisia, parkinsonism, tardive dyskinesia and plasma neuroleptic levels. *Br J Psychiatry* 1992;160:793–9

40. Glazer WM, Morgenstern H, Doucette JT. Predicting the long-term risk of tardive dyskinesia in outpatients maintained on neuroleptic medications. *J Clin Psychiatry* 1993;54:133–9

41. Reilly JG, Ayis SA, Ferrier IN, *et al.* QTc-interval abnormalities and psychotropic drug therapy in psychiatric patients. *Lancet* 2000;355:1048–52

42. Yap YG, Camm J. Risk of torsades de pointes with non-cardiac drugs. Doctors need to be aware that many drugs can cause qt prolongation [Editorial]. *Br Med J* 2000;320:1158–9

43. Morganroth J, Brozovich FV, McDonald JT, Jacobs RA. Variability of the QT measurement in healthy men, with implications for selection of an abnormal QT value to predict drug toxicity and proarrhythmia. *Am J Cardiol* 1991;67:774–6

44. Schoemaker H, Claustre Y, Fage D, *et al.* Neurochemical characteristics of amisulpride, an atypical dopamine D2/D3 receptor antagonist with both presynaptic and limbic selectivity. *J Pharmacol Exp Ther* 1997;280:83–97

45. Schotte A, Janssen PF, Gommeren W. *et al.* Risperidone compared with new and reference antipsychotic drugs: *in vitro* and *in vivo* receptor binding. *Psychopharmacology* 1996;124:57–73

46. Travis MJ. Clozapine. A review. *J Serotonin Res* 1997;4:125–44

47. Kane J, Honigfeld G, Singer J, Meltzer H. Clozapine for the treatment-resistant schizophrenic: a double blind comparison with chlorpromazine. *Arch Gen Psychiatry* 1988;45:789–96

48. Claghorn J, Honigfeld G, Abuzzahab FS Sr, *et al.* The risks and benefits of clozapine versus chlorpromazine. *J Clin Psychopharmacol* 1987;7:377–84

49. Conley RR, Schulz SC, Baker RW, *et al.* Clozapine efficacy in schizophrenic nonresponders. *Psychopharmacol Bull* 1988;24:269–74

50. Breier A, Buchanan RW, Waltrip RWI, *et al.* The effects of clozapine on plasmanorepinephrine: relationship to clinical efficacy. *Neuropsychopharmacology* 1994;10:1–7

51. Pickar D, Owen RR, Litman RE, *et al.* Clinical and biologic response to clozapine in patients with schizophrenia. Crossover comparison with fluphenazine [see comments]. *Arch Gen Psychiatry* 1992;49: 345–53

52. Essock SM, Hargreaves WA, Covell NH, Goethe J. Clozapine's effectiveness for patients in state hospitals: results from a randomized trial. *Psychopharmacol Bull* 1996;32:683–97

53. Marder SR, Davis JM, Chouinard G. The effects of risperidone on the five dimensions of schizophrenia derived by factor analysis: combined results of the North American trials. *J Clin Psychiatry* 1997;58: 538–46

54 Song F. Risperidone in the treatment of schizophrenia: a meta-analysis of randomized controlled trials. *J Psychopharmacol* 1997;11:65–71

55. Overall JE, Gorham DR. The Brief Psychiatric Rating Scale. *Psychological Reports* 1962;10:799–812

56. Tollefson GD, Sanger TM. Negative symptoms: a path analytic approach to a double-blind, placebo- and haloperidol-controlled clinical trial with olanzapine. *Am J Psychiatry* 1997;154:466–74

57. Dellva MA, Tran P, Tollefson GD, *et al.* Standard olanzapine versus placebo and ineffective-dose olanzapine in the maintenance treatment of schizophrenia [see comments]. *Psychiatric Serv* 1997;48: 1571–7

58. Small JG, Hirsch SR, Arvanitis LA, *et al.* Quetiapine in patients with schizophrenia. A high- and low-dose double-blind comparison with placebo. Seroquel Study Group. *Arch Gen Psychiatry* 1997;54:549–57

59. Peuskens J, Link CG. A comparison of quetiapine and chlorpromazine in the treatment of schizophrenia. *Acta Psychiatr Scand* 1997;96:265–73

60. Arvanitis LA, Miller BG. Multiple fixed doses of 'Seroquel' (quetiapine) in patients with acute exacerbation of schizophrenia: a comparison with haloperidol and placebo. The Seroquel Trial 13 Study Group. *Biol Psychiatry* 1997;42:233–46

61. Rak IW, Jone AM, Raniwalla J, *et al.* Weight changes in patients treated with seroquel (quetiapine). *Schizophrenia Res* 2000;41(special issue):206

62. Hellewell JSE, Kalali AH, Langham SJ, McKellar J, Awad AG. Patient satisfaction and acceptability of long-term treatment with quetiapine. *Int J Psychiatry Clin Pract* 1999;3:105–13

63. Xiberas X, Martinot JL, Mallet L, *et al.* In vivo extrastriatal and striatal D2 dopamine receptor blockade by amisulpride in schizophrenia. *J Clin Psychopharmacol* 2001;21:207

64. Delcker A, Schoon ML, Oczkowski B, Gaertner HJ. Amisulpride versus haloperidol in treatment of schizophrenic patients – results of a double-blind study. *Pharmacopsychiatry* 1990;23:125–30

65. Moller HJ, Boyer P, Fleurot O, Rein W. Improvement of acute exacerbations of schizophrenia with amisulpride: a comparison with haloperidol. PROD-ASLP Study Group. *Psychopharmacology* 1997;132: 396–401

66. Puech A, Fleurot O, Rein W. Amisulpride, and atypical antipsychotic, in the treatment of acute episodes of schizophrenia: a dose-ranging study vs. haloperidol. The Amisulpride Study Group. *Acta Psychiatr Scand* 1998;98:65–72

67. Carriere P, Bonhomme D, Lemperiere T. Amisulpride has a superior benefit/risk profile to haloperidol in schizophrenia: results of a multi-centre, double-blind study (the Amisulpride Study Group). *Eur Psychiatry* 2000;15:321–9

68. Coulouvrat C, Dondey-Nouvel L. Safety of amisulpride (Solian): a review of 11 clinical studies. *Int Clin Psychopharmacol* 1999;14:209–18

69. Rein W, Coulouvrat C, Dondey-Nouvel L. Safety profile of amisulpride in short- and long-term use. *Acta Psychiatr Scand* 2000;400(Suppl.):23–7

70. Colonna L, Saleem P, Dondey-Nouvel L, Rein W. Long-term safety and efficacy of amisulpride in sub-chronic or chronic schizophrenia. Amisulpride Study Group. *Int Clin Psychopharmacol* 2000;15:13–22

71. Goff DC, Posever T, Herz L, *et al.* An exploratory haloperidol-controlled dose-finding study of ziprasidone in hospitalized patients with schizophrenia or schizoaffective disorder. *J Clin Psychopharmacol* 1998;18:296–304

72. Keck P, Jr, Buffenstein A, Ferguson J, *et al.* Ziprasidone 40 and 120 mg/day in the acute exacerbation of schizophrenia and schizoaffective disorder: a 4-week placebo-controlled trial. *Psychopharmacology* 1998;140:173–84

73. Daniel DG, Zimbroff DL, Potkin SG, *et al.* Ziprasidone 80 mg/day and 160 mg/day in the acute exacerbation of schizophrenia and schizoaffective disorder: a 6-week placebo-controlled trial. Ziprasidone Study Group. *Neuropsychopharmacology* 1999; 20:491–505

74. Arato M, O'Connor R, Meltzer H, *et al.* The ziprasidone extended use in schizophrenia (ZEUS) study: a propective, double blind, placebo controlled, 1 year clinical trial. *Data on file, Pfizer Pharmaceutical Group,* 1999

75. Corbett R, Griffiths L, Shipley JE, *et al.* Iloperidone: Preclinical profile and early clinical evaluation. *CNS Drug Reviews* 1997;3:120–47

76. Jain KK. An assessment of iloperidone for the treatment of schizophrenia. *Exp Opin Invest Drugs* 2000;9:2935–43

77. Cucchiaro J, Nann-Vernotica E, Lasser R, *et al.* A randomised double-blind, multicenter phase II study of iloperidone versus haloperidole and placebo in patients with schizophrenia or schizoaffective disorder. *Schizophr Res* 2001;49:223

78. Lawler CP, Prioleau C, Lewis MM, *et al.* Interactions of the novel antipsychotic aripiprazole (OPC-14597) with dopamine and serotonin receptor subtypes. *Neuropsychopharmacology* 1999;20:612–27

79. Petrie JL, Saha AR, Ali MW. Safety and efficacy profile of aripiprazole, a novel antipsychotic. *Presented at the 37th Annual ACNP Meeting*

80. Carson WH, Ali M, Saha A, *et al.* A double-blind placebo controlled trial of aripiprazole and haloperidol. *Schizophrenia Res* 2001;49(Suppl. 1–2):221–2

81. Lieberman JA, Saltz BL, Johns CA, *et al.* The effects of clozapine on tardive dyskinesia. *Br J Psychiatry* 1991;158:503–10

82. Gerlach J, Peacock L. Motor and mental side effects of clozapine. *J Clin Psychiatry* 1994;55(Suppl. B): 107–9

83. Tamminga CA, Thaker GK, Moran M, *et al.* Clozapine in tardive dyskinesia: observations for human and animal model studies. *J Clin Psychiatry* 1994;55(Suppl B):102–6

84. Shapleske J, Mickay AP, Mckenna PJ. Successful treatment of tardive dystonia with clozapine and clonazepam. *Br J Psychiatry* 1996;168:516–18

85. Jibson MD, Tandon R. New atypical antipsychotic medications. *J Psychiatric Res* 1998;32:215–28

86. Meltzer HY. Pharmacologic treatment of negative symptoms. In Greden JF, Tandon R, eds. *Negative Schizophrenic Symptoms: Pathophysiology and Clinical Implications.* Washington, DC: American Psychiatric Press, 1990:215–31

87. Tandon R, Ribeiro SC, DeQuardo JR, *et al.* Covariance of positive and negative symptoms during neuroleptic treatment in schizophrenia: a replication. *Biol Psychiatry* 1993;34:495–7

88. Hagger C, Buckley P, Kenny JT, *et al.* Improvement in cognitive functions and psychiatric symptoms in treatment refractory schizophrenic patients receiving clozapine. *Biol Psychiatry* 1993;34:702–12

89. Breier A, Buchanan RW, Kirkpatrick B, *et al.* Effects of clozapine on positive and negative symptoms in outpatients with schizophrenia. *Am J Psychiatry* 1994;151:20–6

90. Conley R, Gounaris C, Tamminga C. Clozapine response varies in deficit versus non-deficit schizophrenic subjects. *Biol Psychiatry* 1994;35:746–7

91. Kane JM, Safferman AZ, Pollack S, *et al.* Clozapine, negative symptoms, and extrapyramidal side effects. *J Clin Psychiatry* 1994;55(9, suppl B):74–7

92. Carpenter WT Jr. Maintainence therapy of persons with schizophrenia. *J Clin Psychiatry* 1996;57 (Suppl. 9):10–18

93. Tollefson GD, Beasley CM Jr, Tran PV, Street JS. Olanzapine versus haloperidol in the treatment of schizophrenia and schizoaffective and schizophreniform disorders: results of an international collaborative trial [see comments]. *Am J Psychiatry* 1997;154:457–65

94. Danion JM, Rein W, Fleurot O. Improvement of schizophrenic patients with primary negative symptoms treated with amisulpride. Amisulpride Study Group. *Am J Psychiatry* 1999;156:610–6

95. Boyer P, Lecrubier Y, Puech AJ, *et al.* Treatment of negative symptoms in schizophrenia with amisulpride. *Br J Psychiatry* 1995;166:68–72

96. Paillere-Martinot ML, Lecrubier Y, Martinot JL, Aubin F. Improvement of some schizophrenic deficit symptoms with low doses of amisulpride. *Am J Psychiatry* 1995;152:130–4

97. Speller JC, Barnes TR, Curson DA, *et al.* One-year, low-dose neuroleptic study of in-patients with chronic schizophrenia characterised by persistent negative symptoms. Amisulpride v. haloperidol. *Br J Psychiatry* 1997;171:564–8

98. Meltzer HY, Thompson PA, Lee MA, Ranjan R. Neuropsychologic deficits in schizophrenia: relation to social function and effect of antipsychotic drug treatment. *Neuropsychopharmacology* 1996;14(Suppl 3):27S–33S

99. Bilder RM. Neurocognitive impairment in schizophrenia and how it affects treatment options. *Can J Psychiatry – Revue Can Psychiatrie* 1997;42: 255–64

100. Lee MA, Thompson PA, Meltzer HY. Effects of clozapine on cognitive function in schizophrenia. [Review]. *J Clin Psychiatry* 1994;55(Suppl B):82–7

101. Gallhofer B, Bauer U, Lis S, *et al.* Cognitive dysfunction in schizophrenia:comparison of treatment with atypical antipsychotic agents and conventional neuroleptic drugs. *Eur Neuropsychopharmacol* 1996;6(Suppl. 2):S13–20

102. Green MF, Marshall BD, Jr., Wirshing WC, *et al.* Does risperidone improve verbal working memory in treatment-resistant schizophrenia? *Am J Psychiatry* 1997;154:799–804

103. McGurk SR, Meltzer HY. The effects of atypical antipsychotic drugs on cognitive functioning in schizophrenia. *Schizophrenia Res* 1998;29:160

104. Sax KW, Strakowski SM, Keck PE Jr. Attentional improvement following quetiapine fumarate treatment in schizophrenia. *Schizophr Res* 1998;33:151–5

105. Peretti CS, Danion JM, Kauffmann-Muller F, *et al.* Effects of haloperidol and amisulpride on motor and cognitive skill learning in healthy volunteers. *Psychopharmacology* 1997;131:329–38

106. Zarate CAJ, Tohen M, Banov MD, *et al.* Is clozapine a mood stabilizer? *J Clin Psychiatry* 1995;56:108–12

107. Kimmel SE, Calabrese JR, Woyshville MJ, Meltzer HY. Clozapine in treatment-refractory mood disorders [Review]. *J Clin Psychiatry* 1994;55(Suppl B):91–3

108. Calabrese JR, Kimmel SE, Woyshville MJ, *et al.* Clozapine for treatment-refractory mania. *Am J Psychiatry* 1996;156:759–64

109. Meltzer HY, Okayli G. Reduction of suicidality during clozapine treatment of neuroleptic-resistant schizophrenia: impact on risk benefit assessment. *Am J Psychiatry* 1995;152:183–90

110. Banov MD, Zarate CAJ, Tohen M, *et al.* Clozapine therapy in refractory affective disorders: polarity predicts response in long term follow up. *J Clin Psychiatry* 1994;55:295–300

111. Rothschild AJ. Management of psychotic, treatment resistant depression. *Psychiatr Clin North Am* 1996; 19:237–52

112. Tollefson GD, Sanger TM, Lu Y, Thieme ME. Depressive signs and symptoms in schizophrenia: a prospective blinded trial of olanzapine and haloperidol [published erratum appears in *Arch Gen Psychiatry* 1998;55:1052]. *Arch Gen Psychiatry* 1998;55:250–8

113. Lecrubier Y, Boyer P, Turjanski S, Rein W. Amisulpride versus imipramine and placebo in dysthymia and major depression. Amisulpride Study Group. *J Affect Dis* 1997;43:95–103

114. Geddes J, Freemantle N, Harrison P, Bebbington P. Atypical antipsychotics in the treatment of schizophrenia: systematic overview and meta-regression analysis. [see comments]. *Br Med J* 2000;321:1371–6

115. Kapur S, Remington G. Atypical antipsychotics. [letter]. *Br Med J* 2000;321:1360–1

116. Prior C, Clements J, Rowett M, *et al.* Atypical antipsychotics in the treatment of schizophrenia. *Br Med J* 2001;322:924

117. Taylor, D. Low dose typical antipsychotics – a brief evaluation. *Psychiatr Bull* 2000;24:465–8

118. Arranz MJ, Munro J, Birkett J, *et al.* Pharmacogenetic prediction of clozapine response. *Lancet* 2000;355: 1615–6

CHAPTER 5

Psychosocial management

It is obvious that the successful management of schizophrenia requires careful attention to much more than just pharmacology. All good clinicians spend a large proportion of their time dealing with issues that can broadly be described as 'psychosocial'. However, because it is very difficult to distill the relevant psychosocial issues down to a set of rigorously evaluable interventions, this important aspect of treatment is under-researched and relatively unacknowledged. Research into specific areas of psychosocial management falls into two main categories: the effectiveness of individual psychological therapies, and the optimal organization of mental health services. Research in both areas suffers from the perennial methodological difficulties of adequate control groups and statistical power, and from questions over the extent to which one can generalize from small research settings to large-scale clinical implementation. Nevertheless, psychosocial interventions have become increasingly prominent components of health policy[1].

PSYCHOLOGICAL THERAPIES

Psychoanalytic psychotherapies have largely been discredited in the management of schizophrenia, and indeed cast something of a shadow over the development of more effective approaches to treatment. However, a number of very promising new approaches are now emerging.

Cognitive behavioral therapy

Cognitive behavioral therapy (CBT) encompasses a variety of interventions. At its core is the idea that if patients can be presented with a credible 'cognitive' model of their symptoms, they may develop more adaptive coping strategies, leading to reduced distress, improved social function and possibly even symptom reduction. CBT involves regular one-to-one contact over a defined time period between patient and therapist, the latter often (but not always) a clinical psychologist (other professionals including community psychiatric nurses and psychiatrists are becoming increasingly involved as trained therapists) (Figure 5.1). The treatment packages emphasize engagement and insight, and devote considerable

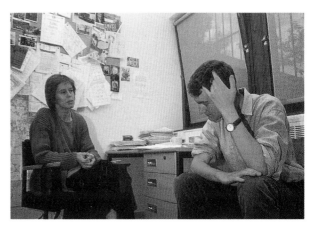

Figure 5.1 Professor Elizabeth Kuipers, one of the pioneers of cognitive behavioral therapy (CBT) for psychosis, treating a 'patient' [played here by a colleague]

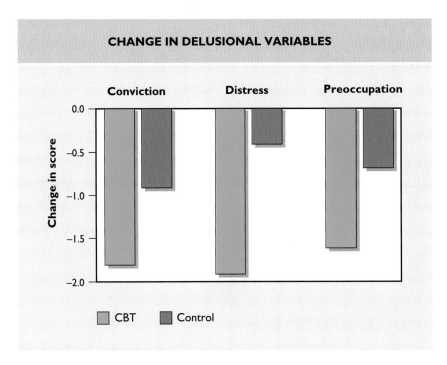

CHANGE IN DELUSIONAL VARIABLES

Figure 5.2 Sixty patients with chronic schizophrenia were randomized to nine months of cognitive behavioral therapy (CBT) and standard care, or standard care alone. At 18 months, patients with delusions who had received CBT were found to hold these with a reduced level of conviction, and were less preoccupied and distressed by their delusional beliefs. Figure reproduced with permission from Kuipers E, Garety P, Fowler D, et al. The London-East Anglia randomised controlled trial of cognitive-behavioural therapy for psychosis: III. Follow-up and economic evaluation at 18 months. Br J Psychiatry 173:61–8

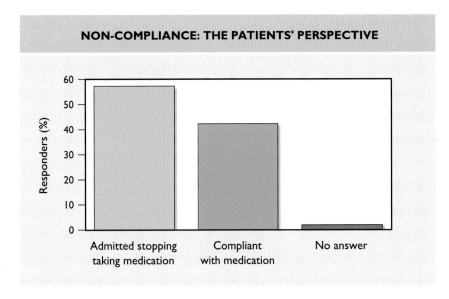

NON-COMPLIANCE: THE PATIENTS' PERSPECTIVE

Figure 5.3 Over half of a group of 615 patients admitted to having stopped their medication. Figure reproduced with kind permission from Hellewell, JSE. Antipsychotic tolerability: the attitudes and perceptions of medical professionals, patients and caregivers towards the side effects of antipsychotic therapy. Euro Neuropsychopharmacol 1998;8:S248

attention to agreeing a common therapeutic agenda. Relatively non-specific elements form an important component of all treatment packages, including basic information about schizophrenia and its drug treatment, strategies to manage associated anxiety and depression, and interventions to tackle negative symptoms and social function. More specific strategies to target positive symptoms include formulating, together with the

patient, alternative, more adaptive explanatory models for delusions and hallucinations.

There are, however, substantial differences of detail between published studies, for example with respect to the duration of the intervention, or the incorporation of family work. A distinction is also made between CBT for acute and for chronic schizophrenia, although results are encouraging in both contexts (Figure 5.2)[2–5]. However, at the

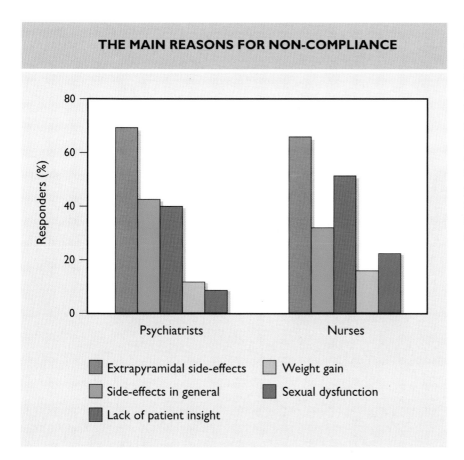

Figure 5.4 The views of psychiatrists and nurses on the main reasons for patients' non-compliance with medication. Both groups underestimate the importance of sexual side-effects, the psychiatrists more so than the nurses. Figure reproduced with kind permission from Hellewell, JSE. Antipsychotic tolerability: the attitudes and perceptions of medical professionals, patients and caregivers towards the side effects of antipsychotic therapy. *Euro Neuropsychopharmacol* 1998;8:S248

time of writing, the published data do not exclude the possibility that many of the beneficial effects may arise from non-specific factors, such as befriending and increased contact time with the therapist.

Neurocognitive remediation

Neurocognitive remediation attempts to improve cognitive function, and thereby influence symptoms and functional outcome for the better through task practise and repetition. Cognitive function is a key determinant of long-term outcome in schizophrenia[6], but to date, the clinical results of interventions focusing on specific cognitive deficits have been disappointing. At a more practical level, vocational rehabilitation and social skills training remain important elements of many treatment programmes with a focus on rehabilitation and functional outcome.

Compliance with drug treatment

This is another important determinant of outcome in schizophrenia, since the majority of patients admit to stopping their medication at some stage (Figure 5.3). The latter is hardly surprising, since they are asked to take drugs with unpleasant side-effects, including extrapyramidal symptoms, weight gain and sexual dysfunction (Figure 5.4) for long periods of time. Few psychiatrists stop to think whether they themselves would be 100% compliant in taking regular medication in the face of such side-effects. Compliance therapy[7] uses simple psychological interventions focusing on the psychological aspects of long-term drug treatment in schizophrenia, emphasising insight and the formation of a therapeutic alliance between prescriber and patient, and appears to be effective and relatively straightforward to incorporate into routine practice.

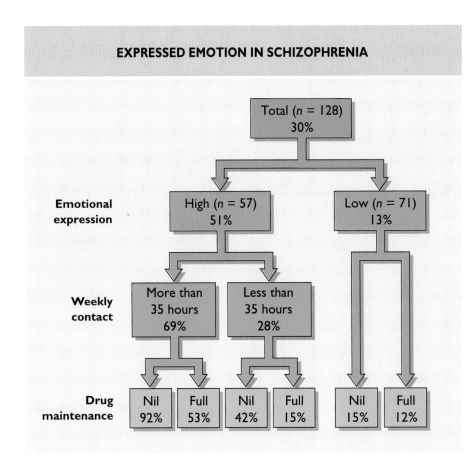

EXPRESSED EMOTION IN SCHIZOPHRENIA

Total (n = 128)
30%

Emotional expression

High (n = 57)
51%

Low (n = 71)
13%

Weekly contact

More than 35 hours
69%

Less than 35 hours
28%

Drug maintenance

| Nil | Full | Nil | Full | Nil | Full |
| 92% | 53% | 42% | 15% | 15% | 12% |

Figure 5.5 This figure shows the results of a trial of maintenance antipsychotics in patients divided according to whether their families showed high expressed emotion (EE) or not. The degree of EE in families predicts relapse in patients with schizophrenia who are not taking antipsychotic drugs, and who are in contact with their familites for more than 35 hours each week

Family treatments

It has long been recognised that high levels of 'expressed emotion' (EE) in the family increase the risk of relapse in unmedicated patients (Figure 5.5). The question then arose whether psychological interventions with the families of schizophrenic patients might have any effect on this. Family therapy in schizophrenia is based on a 'psycho-educational' approach which includes information about the nature of the disorder, its treatment, and factors (including EE) which might modify its course. It appears to have a modest effect in reducing the risk of relapse in schizophrenia[8], although this may not in fact be directly mediated through a specific effect on EE. Another important source of family input exists in the voluntary sector, where groups such as (in the UK) the National Schizophrenia Fellowship can be extremely helpful in providing support and information for the relatives and carers of people with schizophrenia.

Early intervention

Much interest has recently focused on the treatment of schizophrenia early in the first episode of illness. The impetus behind this is preventative: many studies have shown a mean duration of untreated psychosis of the order of one year. Underlying this is a bimodal distribution: people with florid psychosis often present fairly rapidly, particularly if their symptoms bring them into conflict with families or wider society, but others with more insiduously-developing illnesses can take many years to come to psychiatric attention. It is argued that the early stages of illness represent an opportunity for intervention which may modify its long-term course and minimize the degree of residual disability[9]. For early intervention to succeed, the repertoire of psychosocial interventions in schizophrenia must include public education, improving referral pathways from primary care, and challenging stigmatizing and discriminatory attitudes to people with

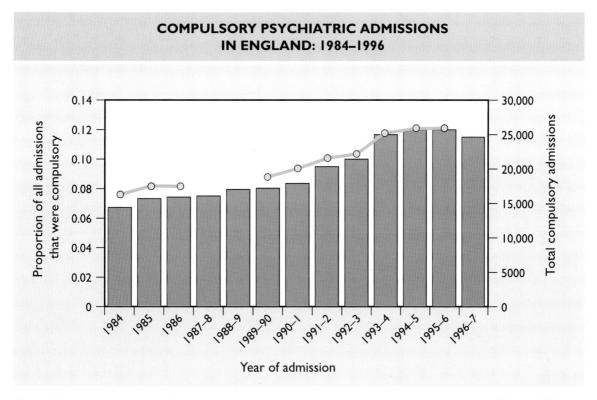

**COMPULSORY PSYCHIATRIC ADMISSIONS
IN ENGLAND: 1984–1996**

Figure 5.6 Despite the policy of care in the community there was a rise in total admissions between 1984 and 1996, and a rise in the proportion of compulsory admissions. A combination of increased prevalence of comorbid drug misuse, reductions in available bed numbers (a reduction of 43 000 in the UK between 1982 and 1992), and changes in the thresholds for admission and discharge, has meant that patients are more severely ill before admission, and services are under greater pressure, leading to a paradoxical increase in the use of compulsory detention. (Bars represent the total number of compulsory psychiatric admissions to NHS facilities and the line represents the proportion of all admissions that were compulsory in England, 1984–96. Data on compulsory admissions not available for 1987–89). Figure reproduced with permission from Wall S, Hotopf M, Wessely S, Churchill R. Trends in the use of the Mental Health Act, England 1984–1996. *Br Med J* 1999;318:1520–1

schizophrenia which act as disincentives to early referral and treatment.

Managing schizophrenia in the community

The move toward treating people with schizophrenia in the community (Figures 1.15 and 5.6) was made possible (both clinically and politically), from the 1950s onwards, by the introduction of effective antipsychotic drugs. The purpose of this was to give patients with psychosis a better quality of life, and there is no doubt that patients generally prefer to be treated in their own home rather than in hospital (Figure 5.7). However, since drug treatment was so crucial to the move towards community care, the delivery and monitoring of

medication became a major preoccupation of the organizational systems that developed to support it. A second priority, intermittently reinforced by clinical scandal and catastrophe, has been the assessment and management of the risks, both perceived and real, associated with the shift of care away from the relatively secure and contained environment of the hospital ward. Thirdly, the new community mental health teams needed to lubricate the interactions between their ill and sometimes institutionalized patients and the complex bureaucracies – housing, social security, the judicial system, employers – of the outside world. However, none of this should distract us from the objective of delivering better care, and the awareness that good care involves more than simply drug treatment.

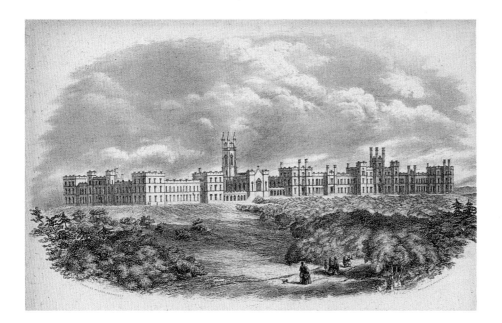

Figure 5.7 Prior to the 1950s and the introduction of effective antipsychotic treatment, most patients with schizophrenia would have been institutionalized in large-scale psychiatric hospitals. This painting from 1843 shows one such hospital in Gartnavel, Glasgow, UK

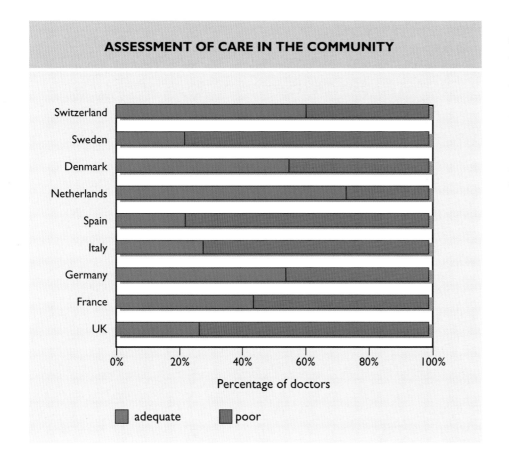

ASSESSMENT OF CARE IN THE COMMUNITY

Percentage of doctors

■ adequate   ■ poor

Figure 5.8 An international study of pyschiatrists' attitudes to community care. Note that the countries in which psychiatrists have the most positive attitudes, Switzerland, Denmark, The Netherlands and Germany, have the highest per capita spending on mental health services.

Various models have evolved in the face of these demands. These are mostly based on variations of 'case management', in which mental health workers take responsibility for the planning, co-ordination, review, and to varying extents the delivery of care 'packages' to individual patients. In practise, most services organized on these principles have developed eclectic and pragmatic ways of working, which have proved at least as effective as more hospital-based models of clinical care[10]. The formal models differ in their specifics, for example in the precise role of the keyworker, caseload, organizational philosophy, and specialist functions, such as assertive outreach and crisis intervention. The benefit of one approach over any other remains a matter of debate (see for example reference 11). In any event, such organizational models should not be confused with treatments, and their clinical impact on specific symptoms is likely to be indirect and less pronounced than their effect on more general social variables such as housing stability. Comparisons between different approaches to the organization of community psychiatric care are made more difficult by wide variations internationally in clinical practice and in resources, and there are wide international differences in the extent to which community care is regarded as a successful policy (Figure 5.8)[14].

REFERENCES

1. Hemsley D, Murray RM. Psychological and social treatments for schizophrenia: not just old remedies in new bottles. *Schizophr Bull* 2000;26:145–51

2. Drury V, Birchwood M, Cochrane R, MacMillan F. Cognitive therapy and recovery from acute psychosis: I. Impact on symptoms. *Br J Psychiatry* 1996; 169:593–601

3. Drury V, Birchwood M, Cochrane R, MacMillan F. Cognitive therapy and recovery from acute psychosis: II. Impact on recovery time. *Br J Psychiatry* 1996;169:602–7

4. Kuipers E, Garety P, Fowler D, *et al*. The London-East Anglia randomised controlled trial of cognitive-behavioural therapy for psychosis: III. Follow-up and economic evaluation at 18 months. *Br J Psychiatry* 1998;173:61–8

5. Tarrier N, Yusupoff L, *et al*. Randomised controlled trial of intensive cognitive behaviour therapy for patients with chronic schizophrenia. *Br Med J* 1998; 317:303–7

6. Green MF. What are the functional consequences of neurocognitive deficits in schizophrenia? *Am J Psychiatry* 1996;153:321–30

7. Kemp R, Hayward P, *et al*. Compliance therapy in psychotic patients: a randomised controlled trial. *Br Med J* 1996;312:345–9

8. Pharoah FM, Mari JJ, Streiner D. Family intervention for schizophrenia (Cochrane Review). In *The Cochrane Library*. Oxford: Update Software, 1999: issue 3

9. Birchwood M, Todd P, Jackson C. Early intervention in psychosis: the critical-period hypothesis. *Int Clin Psychopharm* 1998;13(Suppl 1):S31–S40

10. Tyrer P, Coid J, Simmonds S, *et al*. Community mental health teams for people with severe mental illnesses and disordered personality (Cochrane Review). In *The Cochrane Library*. Oxford: Update Software, 1999:issue 3

11. Burns T, Creed F, *et al*. Intensive versus standard case management for severe psychotic illness: a randomised trial. *Lancet* 1999;353:2185–9

12. Mueser KT, Bond GR, Drake RE, Resnick SG. Models of community care for severe mental illness: a review of research on case management. *Schizophr Bull* 1998;24:37–74

13. Wall S, Hotopf M, Wessely S, Churchill R. Trends in the use of the Mental Health Act, England 1984-1996. *Br Med J* 1999;318:1520–1

14. Smith-Latten, Grimdy S. *Survey of European Psychiatrists*. London: Martin Hamlyn

Index